HOW TO STOP SNORING

Josh C. Pete

COPYRIGHT PAGE © 2024

All rights reserved. No part of this publication may be reproduced, distributed, or transmitted in any form or by any means, including photocopying, recording, or other electronic or mechanical methods, without the prior written permission of the author, except in the case of brief quotations embodied in critical reviews and certain other non-commercial uses permitted by copyright law.

Table Of Contents

Introduction 5
- Understanding Snoring 5
- What Causes Snoring? 8
- How Snoring Affects Your Health 10
- Different Types of Snoring 15

Assessing Your Snoring 20
- Recognizing the Severity of Your Snoring 20
- Keeping a Snoring Diary 24
- Seeking Medical Evaluation 29

Lifestyle Changes 35
- Improving Sleep Hygiene 35
- Establishing a Consistent Sleep Schedule 40
- Creating a Relaxing Bedtime Routine 46
- Optimizing Your Sleep Environment 51

Healthy Eating Habits for Better Sleep 58
- Foods That Can Aggravate Snoring 58
- Snoring-Friendly Diet Tips 63
- The Role of Weight Management 68

Avoiding Alcohol and Sedatives 73
- Understanding the Effects of Alcohol on Sleep 73
- Identifying Sedatives That Can Worsen Snoring ..78
- Strategies for Reducing Dependency on Sleep Aids 83

Practical Techniques 88
- Positional Therapy 88
    - Sleeping Positions That Reduce Snoring 90
    - Using Pillows and Wedges for Positional Therapy 94
    - Training Yourself to Sleep in a Preferred

Position 98
- Nasal Congestion Relief 102
   - Identifying Nasal Congestion Triggers 102
   - Home Remedies for Clearing Nasal Passages107
   - Using Nasal Strips and Sprays Effectively...111
- Throat and Tongue Exercises 117
   - Strengthening Exercises for Throat Muscles117
   - Tongue Exercises to Prevent Obstruction ...121
   - Incorporating Daily Exercise Routines 125

Devices and Medical Treatments............................131
- Oral Appliances for Snoring................................134
- How Mandibular Advancement Devices Work ...138
- Choosing the Right Oral Appliance 143
- Adjusting to Using Oral Appliances 148

Continuous Positive Airway Pressure (CPAP)
Therapy 153
- Understanding CPAP Machines and Masks 153
- Overcoming Common CPAP Challenges...........157
- CPAP Alternatives and Variations 165

Surgical Options for Snoring 170
- Types of Surgical Procedures Available:............171
- Risks and Benefits of Surgical Intervention:.......172
- Considering Surgery as a Last Resort:...............173

Seeking Professional Help 174
- Consulting with Sleep Specialists.......................176
- Participating in Sleep Studies.............................179
- Exploring Advanced Treatment Options.............183

Coping Strategies for Partners 188
- Understanding the Impact of Snoring on
Relationships 189
- Communication Techniques for Addressing
Snoring Concerns 192
- Seeking Support and Resources for Partners....196

Long-Term Maintenance and Prevention............200
- Monitoring Snoring Patterns Over Time.............201
- Incorporating Healthy Habits into Your Lifestyle 204
- Staying Informed about Advances in Snoring Treatment...207
Conclusion..**212**

Introduction

- *Understanding Snoring*

Understanding snoring requires a grasp of its underlying causes and mechanisms. Snoring occurs when the flow of air through the mouth and nose is partially obstructed during sleep, causing vibrations of the soft tissues in the upper airway. These vibrations produce the familiar sound of snoring. Various factors contribute to this obstruction, including the relaxation of throat muscles, narrowing of the airway due to anatomical factors like enlarged tonsils or adenoids, and congestion in the nasal passages.

One common cause of snoring is poor sleep posture. When sleeping on the back, the tongue and soft tissues of the throat can collapse backward, obstructing the airway and leading to snoring. Additionally, excess weight, particularly around the neck and throat area, can exacerbate snoring by putting pressure on the airway. Lifestyle factors such as alcohol consumption and smoking can also contribute to snoring by relaxing throat muscles and causing inflammation in the airway.

Understanding the types of snoring can provide insight into its severity and potential health implications. Primary snoring, characterized by noisy breathing during sleep without associated pauses in breathing or arousal, is generally considered benign. However, habitual snoring, especially when accompanied by other symptoms such as daytime sleepiness or witnessed pauses in breathing, may indicate a more serious condition known as obstructive sleep apnea (OSA). OSA occurs when the airway becomes completely blocked during sleep, leading to repeated episodes of interrupted breathing and disrupted sleep.

It's essential to recognize that snoring is not just a nuisance but can also have significant health consequences. Chronic snoring and untreated sleep apnea have been linked to a range of health issues, including high blood pressure, heart disease, stroke, and cognitive impairment. Furthermore, snoring can disrupt the sleep of both the snorer and their sleeping partner, leading to daytime fatigue, irritability, and strained relationships.

To effectively address snoring, it's crucial to undergo a comprehensive evaluation to determine its cause and severity. This may involve keeping a sleep diary to track snoring patterns, undergoing a physical examination to assess the airway, and possibly undergoing a sleep study to diagnose sleep apnea. Armed with a thorough understanding of snoring and its implications, individuals can explore various treatment options, ranging from lifestyle modifications and positional therapy to medical devices and surgical interventions, to improve their sleep quality and overall health.

- What Causes Snoring?

Snoring occurs when the flow of air through the mouth and nose is partially obstructed during sleep, leading to vibrations of the soft tissues in the upper airway. Several factors can contribute to this obstruction:

1. Relaxation of Throat Muscles: During sleep, the muscles in the throat and tongue relax, which can cause them to collapse backward and partially block the airway.

2. Anatomy of the Mouth and Throat: Certain anatomical factors, such as a low, thick soft palate, enlarged tonsils or adenoids, or a long uvula, can narrow the airway and increase the likelihood of snoring.

3. Nasal Congestion: Congestion in the nasal passages due to allergies, sinus infections, or anatomical abnormalities can make it difficult to breathe through the nose, forcing individuals to breathe through their mouth and increasing the risk of snoring.

4. Excess Weight: Being overweight or obese can lead to the accumulation of fatty tissue around the neck and throat, putting pressure on the airway and increasing the likelihood of obstruction during sleep.

5. Sleep Position: Sleeping on the back can cause the tongue and soft tissues in the throat to collapse backward, obstructing the airway and resulting in snoring.

6. Alcohol and Sedatives: Consuming alcohol or certain medications before bedtime can relax the muscles in the throat and tongue, making them more likely to collapse and cause snoring.

7. Age: As people age, the muscles in the throat and tongue may weaken, increasing the likelihood of airway collapse and snoring.

8. Gender: Men are more likely than women to snore, possibly due to differences in anatomy and muscle tone in the upper airway.

Understanding these contributing factors can help individuals identify the potential causes of their snoring and explore appropriate treatment options to address it.

- How Snoring Affects Your Health

Snoring is often dismissed as a mere nuisance, but its impact on health can be significant and far-reaching. Understanding how snoring affects health involves recognizing its association with various physiological and psychological consequences:

1. Sleep Disruption: Snoring disrupts the quality of sleep, not only for the snorer but also for their sleeping partner. The noisy breathing can lead to frequent awakenings throughout the night, preventing individuals from reaching deeper stages of sleep essential for restorative rest. As a result, both the snorer and their partner may experience daytime fatigue, irritability, and difficulty concentrating.

2. Cardiovascular Health: Chronic snoring and its more severe counterpart, obstructive sleep apnea (OSA), have been strongly linked to cardiovascular problems. The repeated episodes of breathing pauses and oxygen deprivation associated with OSA can strain the cardiovascular system, increasing the risk of hypertension (high blood pressure), heart disease, heart attack, and stroke. Additionally, the disrupted sleep patterns caused by snoring may contribute to the development or exacerbation of existing cardiovascular conditions.

3. **Metabolic Health:** Snoring and sleep apnea have been implicated in metabolic disturbances, including insulin resistance and glucose intolerance. These conditions can increase the risk of developing type 2 diabetes and obesity. The fragmented sleep and hormonal imbalances associated with sleep-disordered breathing may disrupt metabolic processes, leading to weight gain and metabolic dysregulation.

4. Neurocognitive Function: Sleep is essential for cognitive function, memory consolidation, and overall brain health. Snoring and sleep apnea can impair cognitive performance and lead to deficits in attention, concentration, and memory. Chronic sleep fragmentation and oxygen desaturation during sleep may contribute to cognitive decline and an increased risk of neurodegenerative conditions such as Alzheimer's disease.

5. Mental Health: The impact of snoring extends beyond physical health to mental well-being. Sleep disturbances caused by snoring can exacerbate or contribute to mood disorders such as depression and anxiety. Sleep-deprived individuals may experience heightened emotional reactivity, mood swings, and reduced stress tolerance. Furthermore, the strain on relationships resulting from disrupted sleep patterns can lead to interpersonal conflicts and negatively affect mental health.

6. **Quality of Life:** Snoring can significantly diminish overall quality of life for both the affected individual and their bed partner. Daytime sleepiness, impaired concentration, and reduced productivity can interfere with work performance and social functioning. Furthermore, the strain on relationships due to sleep disturbances can lead to diminished intimacy, communication difficulties, and overall dissatisfaction with the relationship.

7. **Safety Risks:** Snoring and sleep apnea can pose safety risks, particularly when daytime sleepiness impairs alertness and cognitive function. Individuals with untreated sleep apnea are at an increased risk of motor vehicle accidents and workplace injuries due to impaired vigilance and reaction times.

Understanding the multifaceted impact of snoring on health underscores the importance of addressing this common sleep disorder. Seeking appropriate evaluation and treatment for snoring and sleep apnea can not only improve sleep quality and daytime functioning but also reduce the risk of serious health complications in the long term.

- Different Types of Snoring

Understanding the different types of snoring involves recognizing the various patterns and characteristics of snoring sounds, as well as the underlying factors contributing to each type. While snoring is often generalized as a noisy breathing during sleep, it can manifest in different ways, each indicative of specific anatomical or physiological factors:

1. Primary Snoring: Primary snoring is the most common type and is typically characterized by loud, rhythmic breathing sounds without associated pauses in breathing or arousals from sleep. It occurs when the airflow through the nose and throat is partially obstructed during sleep, leading to vibrations of the soft tissues in the upper airway. While primary snoring may not be associated with significant health risks, it can still disrupt sleep quality and affect the snorer's daytime functioning.

2. Snoring with Mouth Closed: Some individuals may snore primarily with their mouth closed, indicating that the obstruction is occurring predominantly in the nasal passages rather than the throat. This type of snoring may be associated with nasal congestion, deviated septum, or other anatomical abnormalities affecting nasal airflow. Snoring with the mouth closed can be particularly bothersome for the snorer, as it may result in difficulty breathing through the nose during sleep.

3. Snoring with Mouth Open: Conversely, snoring with the mouth open suggests that the obstruction is occurring in the throat or oropharynx. When the muscles in the throat and tongue relax during sleep, they can collapse backward, partially blocking the airway and causing snoring. Sleeping with the mouth open may exacerbate this type of snoring by further narrowing the airway and increasing airflow resistance.

4. **Positional Snoring:** Positional snoring refers to snoring that occurs primarily when the individual is sleeping in a specific position, typically on their back. In this position, gravity pulls the tongue and soft tissues of the throat backward, increasing the likelihood of airway obstruction and snoring. Positional snoring may be alleviated by changing sleep posture or using positional therapy devices, such as special pillows or wearable devices that encourage side sleeping.

5. Snoring with Gasping or Choking Sounds: Snoring accompanied by gasping, choking, or snorting sounds may indicate a more serious condition known as obstructive sleep apnea (OSA). In OSA, the airway becomes completely blocked during sleep, leading to repeated episodes of interrupted breathing and oxygen desaturation. These episodes trigger brief arousals from sleep, often accompanied by gasping or choking sounds as the individual struggles to resume breathing. OSA requires medical evaluation and treatment to prevent complications and improve sleep quality.

6. Snoring in Children: Snoring is not limited to adults and can also occur in children. In pediatric populations, snoring may be associated with conditions such as enlarged tonsils or adenoids, allergies, or anatomical abnormalities affecting the airway.

Chronic snoring in children should be evaluated by a pediatrician or otolaryngologist to rule out underlying causes and prevent potential complications, such as sleep-disordered breathing or developmental issues.

Understanding the different types of snoring can help individuals and healthcare professionals identify the underlying factors contributing to snoring and determine appropriate treatment strategies. Whether primary snoring or indicative of a more serious sleep disorder like sleep apnea, addressing snoring can improve sleep quality, daytime functioning, and overall health and well-being.

Assessing Your Snoring

- Recognizing the Severity of Your Snoring

Recognizing the severity of snoring involves assessing various factors related to the frequency, intensity, and impact of snoring on both the snorer and their sleeping partner. While occasional snoring may be benign, chronic and loud snoring may indicate underlying sleep-disordered breathing or other health concerns. Here's a detailed overview of how to recognize the severity of your snoring:

1. **Frequency and Duration:** Pay attention to how often you snore and how long episodes of snoring last during sleep. Occasional snoring, particularly during times of illness or nasal congestion, may not be cause for concern. However, frequent and persistent snoring most nights of the

week could indicate a more serious problem, especially if it disrupts your sleep or that of your bed partner.

2. Volume and Intensity: Consider the loudness and intensity of your snoring. Loud, disruptive snoring that can be heard from another room or through closed doors may suggest significant airway obstruction or vibration of the soft tissues in the throat. Intense snoring may also be accompanied by gasping, choking, or snorting sounds, which could indicate episodes of obstructive sleep apnea (OSA).

3. Breathing Pauses and Choking Episodes: Take note if your snoring is interrupted by brief pauses in breathing, followed by gasping, choking, or snorting sounds. These episodes, known as apneas, are characteristic of obstructive sleep apnea (OSA) and occur when the airway becomes completely blocked during sleep. If you experience frequent apneas or choking episodes, it's essential to seek medical evaluation for possible sleep apnea.

4. Daytime Symptoms: Consider whether your snoring is accompanied by daytime symptoms such as excessive daytime sleepiness, fatigue, irritability, difficulty concentrating, or morning headaches. These symptoms may indicate that snoring is disrupting your sleep and preventing you from getting restorative rest. Daytime symptoms can significantly impact quality of life and may warrant further evaluation by a healthcare professional.

5. Impact on Bed Partner: Talk to your bed partner or household members about the impact of your snoring on their sleep quality and well-being. Persistent, loud snoring can disrupt your partner's sleep, leading to fatigue, irritability, and strain on the relationship. If your snoring is causing significant disruption to your partner's sleep, it may indicate the need for intervention to address the underlying cause of snoring.

6. Underlying Health Conditions: Consider whether you have any underlying health conditions or risk factors that may contribute to snoring, such as obesity, nasal congestion, allergies, or anatomical abnormalities of the upper airway. Certain medical conditions, medications, or lifestyle factors can exacerbate snoring and increase the risk of sleep-disordered breathing.

7. Self-Assessment Tools: Utilize validated self-assessment tools or questionnaires to evaluate the severity of your snoring and assess your risk of obstructive sleep apnea. These tools may include questions about snoring frequency, daytime symptoms, and other risk factors for sleep apnea. While self-assessment tools can provide useful insights, they are not a substitute for medical evaluation by a healthcare professional.

By considering these factors and recognizing the severity of your snoring, you can make informed decisions about seeking appropriate evaluation and treatment to improve sleep quality, daytime functioning, and overall health and well-being. If you suspect that your snoring may be indicative of a more serious sleep disorder such as obstructive sleep apnea, it's essential to consult with a healthcare professional for further evaluation and management.

- Keeping a Snoring Diary

Keeping a snoring diary can be a valuable tool for understanding the patterns and severity of your snoring, as well as identifying potential triggers and factors that may contribute to snoring episodes. A snoring diary involves recording detailed information about your sleep habits, snoring frequency, and associated symptoms over a period of time. Here's an extensive overview of how to keep a snoring diary:

1. Purpose and Benefits: The primary purpose of a snoring diary is to track and document your snoring patterns and associated symptoms over time. By keeping a detailed record of your sleep habits and snoring episodes, you can identify trends, triggers, and factors that may worsen or alleviate snoring. Additionally, a snoring diary can provide valuable information for healthcare professionals during evaluation and treatment planning for snoring and sleep-related breathing disorders.

2. Recording Sleep Habits: Begin by recording basic information about your sleep habits, including your bedtime, wake-up time, and total duration of sleep each night. Note any deviations from your regular sleep schedule, such as late nights or early mornings, as these may affect your snoring patterns and sleep quality.

3. Snoring Frequency and Intensity: Record the frequency and intensity of your snoring each night. Note whether your snoring occurs intermittently throughout the night or is more persistent and continuous. Use a simple rating scale to describe the loudness or intensity of your snoring, such as mild, moderate, or severe.

4. Sleep Position: Document your sleep position each night, noting whether you sleep on your back, side, or stomach. Positional snoring, which occurs primarily when sleeping on the back, may indicate airway obstruction or relaxation of throat muscles. Tracking sleep position can help identify positional factors contributing to snoring.

5. Associated Symptoms: Record any associated symptoms or sensations experienced during sleep, such as gasping, choking, or snorting sounds, which may indicate episodes of obstructive sleep apnea (OSA). Additionally, note any daytime symptoms such as excessive daytime sleepiness, fatigue, morning headaches, or irritability, which may be related to disrupted sleep from snoring.

6. Environmental Factors: Consider environmental factors that may influence your snoring, such as room temperature, humidity, noise levels, or use of bedding and pillows. Certain environmental conditions, such as dry air or allergens, may exacerbate nasal congestion and contribute to snoring.

7. Lifestyle Factors: Document lifestyle factors that may affect your snoring, such as alcohol consumption, smoking, or use of sedatives or sleep aids. These substances can relax throat muscles and increase the likelihood of airway obstruction during sleep, leading to louder and more persistent snoring.

8. Emotional and Psychological Factors: Consider emotional and psychological factors that may impact your sleep and snoring, such as stress, anxiety, or mood disturbances. Emotional stress and tension can contribute to muscle tension and airway constriction, potentially worsening snoring symptoms.

9. Consistency and Long-Term Tracking: Aim to keep your snoring diary consistently over a period of several weeks or months to capture a comprehensive picture of your snoring patterns and sleep habits. Long-term tracking can help identify fluctuations, trends, and changes in snoring severity over time, as well as assess the effectiveness of interventions or treatments.

By diligently recording information about your sleep habits, snoring patterns, and associated symptoms in a snoring diary, you can gain valuable insights into the factors contributing to your snoring and make informed decisions about lifestyle modifications, treatment options, and when to seek medical evaluation. Additionally, sharing your snoring diary with a healthcare professional can facilitate accurate diagnosis and personalized management of snoring and sleep-related breathing disorders.

- Seeking Medical Evaluation

Seeking medical evaluation for snoring is essential, especially if it is persistent, disruptive, or associated with other symptoms such as daytime sleepiness or gasping episodes during sleep. While occasional snoring may not be cause for concern, chronic and loud snoring can indicate underlying sleep-disordered breathing or other health conditions. Here's an extensive overview of seeking medical evaluation for snoring:

1. **Primary Care Physician:** Start by scheduling an appointment with your primary care physician or general practitioner. Your doctor can assess your snoring symptoms, review your medical history, and perform a physical examination to evaluate potential underlying causes of snoring. Be prepared to discuss details about your sleep habits, snoring patterns, associated symptoms, and any factors that may exacerbate or alleviate your snoring.

2. **Sleep Specialist Referral:** If your primary care physician suspects that your snoring may be indicative of a sleep disorder such as obstructive sleep apnea (OSA), they may refer you to a sleep specialist for further evaluation.

Sleep specialists, typically pulmonologists or otolaryngologists with expertise in sleep medicine, can conduct more comprehensive assessments and diagnostic tests to identify and manage sleep-related breathing disorders.

3. Diagnostic Testing: Depending on the severity and characteristics of your snoring, your healthcare provider may recommend diagnostic tests to evaluate your sleep patterns and breathing during sleep. These tests may include polysomnography (overnight sleep study), home sleep apnea testing (portable monitoring device), or other specialized tests to assess respiratory function and sleep quality.

4. Polysomnography (PSG): Polysomnography is the gold standard diagnostic test for sleep disorders, including obstructive sleep apnea. It involves monitoring various physiological parameters during sleep, such as brain activity, eye movements, muscle tone, heart rate, and breathing patterns. PSG can help determine the presence and severity of sleep apnea, as well as identify other sleep-related abnormalities.

5. Home Sleep Apnea Testing (HSAT): Home sleep apnea testing is a convenient and cost-effective alternative to in-laboratory polysomnography for diagnosing obstructive sleep apnea in select patients with high pretest probability. HSAT typically involves wearing a portable monitoring device overnight at home to measure breathing patterns, oxygen saturation, and other parameters indicative of sleep apnea.

6. Treatment Recommendations: Based on the results of diagnostic testing and evaluation, your healthcare provider can recommend appropriate treatment options to address your snoring and any underlying sleep disorders. Treatment may include lifestyle modifications, positional therapy, oral appliances, continuous positive airway pressure (CPAP) therapy, surgical interventions, or combination therapies tailored to your individual needs and preferences.

7. Follow-Up and Monitoring: After initiating treatment for snoring or sleep-related breathing disorders, it's essential to follow up with your healthcare provider regularly to monitor treatment efficacy, adjust interventions as needed, and address any ongoing concerns or issues. Regular follow-up care ensures optimal management of snoring and associated health conditions, as well as long-term improvements in sleep quality and overall well-being.

By seeking medical evaluation for snoring, you can receive personalized assessment, diagnosis, and treatment recommendations to address your specific sleep-related concerns and improve your quality of life. Don't hesitate to consult with a healthcare professional if you or your bed partner are experiencing persistent or severe snoring, as early intervention can help prevent complications and promote better sleep health.

Lifestyle Changes

- Improving Sleep Hygiene

Improving sleep hygiene involves adopting healthy habits and creating a conducive environment to promote restful and rejuvenating sleep. Sleep hygiene practices aim to optimize sleep quality and quantity by addressing lifestyle factors, bedtime routines, and environmental influences that can affect sleep. Here's an extensive overview of strategies to improve sleep hygiene:

1. Establish a Consistent Sleep Schedule: Go to bed and wake up at the same time every day, even on weekends. Consistency reinforces your body's internal clock, known as the circadian rhythm, and helps regulate sleep-wake cycles. Aim for at least 7-9 hours of sleep per night, depending on your individual needs.

2. Create a Relaxing Bedtime Routine: Develop a calming pre-sleep routine to signal to your body that it's time to wind down and prepare for sleep. This may include activities such as reading a book, taking a warm bath, practicing relaxation techniques (e.g., deep breathing or meditation), or listening to soothing music.

3. Optimize Your Sleep Environment: Create a comfortable and conducive sleep environment that promotes relaxation and restorative sleep. Keep your bedroom cool, quiet, and dark, and minimize exposure to noise, light, and electronic devices that can disrupt sleep. Consider using blackout curtains, earplugs, white noise machines, or sleep masks to enhance sleep quality.

4. Limit Stimulants and Screen Time: Avoid consuming caffeine, nicotine, and other stimulants close to bedtime, as they can interfere with sleep onset and disrupt sleep continuity. Additionally, minimize exposure to electronic screens (e.g., smartphones, tablets, computers) in the hour leading up to bedtime, as the blue light emitted from screens can suppress melatonin production and delay sleep onset.

5. Exercise Regularly: Engage in regular physical activity, but avoid vigorous exercise close to bedtime, as it can increase alertness and delay the onset of sleep. Aim for moderate-intensity exercise earlier in the day, as it can promote better sleep quality and help regulate sleep-wake cycles.

6. Watch Your Diet: Be mindful of your eating habits, particularly in the hours leading up to bedtime. Avoid heavy or spicy meals, large quantities of fluids, and excessive alcohol consumption close to bedtime, as they can disrupt digestion, increase nighttime awakenings, and worsen snoring.

7. Manage Stress and Anxiety: Practice stress-reduction techniques to manage anxiety and promote relaxation before bedtime. This may include mindfulness meditation, progressive muscle relaxation, journaling, or seeking professional support through counseling or therapy if needed.

8. Limit Naps: While short naps can be refreshing and beneficial for some individuals, limit daytime napping to 20-30 minutes and avoid napping late in the day, as it can interfere with nighttime sleep and exacerbate insomnia.

9. Maintain a Comfortable Sleep Environment: Invest in a supportive mattress and pillows that promote proper spinal alignment and comfort during sleep. Choose bedding and sleepwear made from breathable, moisture-wicking materials to help regulate body temperature and minimize discomfort.

10. **Seek Professional Help for Sleep Disorders:** If you experience persistent sleep problems, such as insomnia, sleep apnea, or restless legs syndrome, seek evaluation and treatment from a healthcare professional or sleep specialist. These sleep disorders can significantly impact sleep quality and overall well-being and may require specialized interventions to address.

By incorporating these sleep hygiene practices into your daily routine and creating a conducive sleep environment, you can optimize your sleep quality, promote restful sleep, and enjoy the numerous health benefits associated with adequate and rejuvenating sleep. Experiment with different strategies to find what works best for you, and prioritize sleep as an essential component of your overall health and well-being.

- *Establishing a Consistent Sleep Schedule*

Establishing a consistent sleep schedule is a fundamental aspect of good sleep hygiene and plays a crucial role in regulating your body's internal clock, known as the circadian rhythm. A consistent sleep schedule involves going to bed and waking up at the same time every day, including weekends. Here's an extensive overview of why a consistent sleep schedule is important and how to establish one:

Why Consistency Matters:
1. Regulates Circadian Rhythm: Your body's internal clock, or circadian rhythm, regulates the timing of various physiological processes, including sleep-wake cycles, hormone secretion, and metabolism. Consistent sleep and wake times help synchronize your

circadian rhythm, promoting better sleep quality and overall health.

2. Enhances Sleep Quality: Going to bed and waking up at the same time every day reinforces your body's natural sleep-wake cycle, making it easier to fall asleep and wake up refreshed. Consistent sleep schedules promote deeper, more restorative sleep, reducing the likelihood of sleep disruptions and daytime fatigue.

3. Improves Sleep Efficiency: Consistent sleep schedules optimize sleep efficiency, which refers to the percentage of time spent asleep while in bed. When you maintain a regular sleep schedule, your body learns to anticipate sleep onset and becomes more efficient at transitioning through the various stages of sleep.

4. Stabilizes Hormones and Metabolism: Disruptions to your sleep schedule can affect hormone levels, including cortisol (the stress hormone) and melatonin (the sleep hormone), as well as appetite-regulating hormones such as leptin and ghrelin. Consistent sleep patterns help stabilize hormone secretion and promote metabolic health.

5. Enhances Cognitive Function: Adequate and consistent sleep is essential for cognitive function, memory consolidation, and learning. Following a regular sleep schedule ensures that your brain receives the rest it needs to function optimally, improving attention, concentration, and problem-solving abilities.

Tips for Establishing a Consistent Sleep Schedule:
1. Set a Bedtime and Wake-Up Time: Determine a consistent bedtime and wake-up time that allows for 7-9 hours of sleep per night, depending on your individual sleep needs. Choose a

bedtime that aligns with your natural sleep preferences and lifestyle commitments, and aim to wake up at the same time every day, even on weekends.

2. Gradually Adjust Your Schedule: If you need to shift your sleep schedule, such as when transitioning to a new work schedule or adjusting for daylight saving time, make gradual adjustments over several days to allow your body to adapt gradually. Incrementally adjust your bedtime and wake-up time by 15-30 minutes each day until you reach your desired schedule.

3. Create a Bedtime Routine: Develop a relaxing bedtime routine to signal to your body that it's time to wind down and prepare for sleep. Engage in calming activities such as reading, listening to soothing music, or practicing relaxation techniques like deep breathing or meditation.

4. Limit Exposure to Artificial Light: Minimize exposure to bright artificial light, particularly from electronic screens (e.g., smartphones, tablets, computers), in the hour leading up to bedtime. The blue light emitted from screens can suppress melatonin production and interfere with sleep onset.

5. Optimize Your Sleep Environment: Create a comfortable and conducive sleep environment that promotes relaxation and restorative sleep. Keep your bedroom cool, dark, and quiet, and invest in a supportive mattress and pillows to enhance comfort during sleep.

6. Avoid Stimulants Close to Bedtime: Limit consumption of caffeine, nicotine, and other stimulants in the hours leading up to bedtime, as they can interfere with sleep onset and disrupt sleep quality.

7. Stay Consistent on Weekends: While it may be tempting to sleep in on weekends, try to maintain a consistent sleep schedule by waking up at the same time every day, even on days when you have more flexibility.

8. Monitor Your Sleep Patterns: Keep track of your sleep habits and patterns using a sleep diary or tracking app. Monitoring your sleep can help you identify trends, track progress, and make adjustments as needed to maintain a consistent sleep schedule.

Establishing a consistent sleep schedule requires commitment and discipline, but the benefits to your sleep quality, overall health, and daytime functioning are well worth the effort. By prioritizing sleep consistency and following these tips, you can optimize your sleep-wake cycle, improve sleep quality, and enjoy the numerous benefits of restorative rest.

- Creating a Relaxing Bedtime Routine

Creating a relaxing bedtime routine is essential for winding down after a busy day and preparing your mind and body for restful sleep. A calming bedtime routine can help signal to your body that it's time to transition from wakefulness to sleep, promoting relaxation and improving sleep quality. Here's an extensive overview of how to create a relaxing bedtime routine:

1. Set a Consistent Bedtime: Establish a regular bedtime that allows for 7-9 hours of sleep per night, depending on your individual sleep needs. Consistency reinforces your body's internal clock and helps regulate your sleep-wake cycle.

2. Start Wind-Down Time Early: Begin your bedtime routine at least 30-60 minutes before your intended bedtime to give yourself ample time to relax and unwind before sleep. Avoid engaging in stimulating activities or using electronic devices with bright screens during this time, as they can interfere with melatonin production and delay sleep onset.

3. Dim the Lights: Lower the lights in your home to create a relaxing atmosphere conducive to sleep. Dimming the lights signals to your body that it's time to wind down and prepares you for sleep. Consider using soft, warm-colored lighting in the evening to promote relaxation.

4. Practice Relaxation Techniques: Incorporate relaxation techniques into your bedtime routine to help calm your mind and reduce stress. This may include deep breathing exercises, progressive muscle relaxation, guided imagery, or mindfulness meditation. Experiment with different techniques to find what works best for you.

5. Take a Warm Bath or Shower: A warm bath or shower can help relax tense muscles and soothe your mind, making it easier to fall asleep. Add calming essential oils such as lavender or chamomile to your bathwater to enhance relaxation and promote a sense of calm.

6. Engage in Gentle Stretching or Yoga: Gentle stretching or yoga poses can help release tension in your body and promote relaxation before bedtime. Focus on slow, gentle movements and deep breathing to unwind tight muscles and quiet the mind.

7. Read a Book: Reading a book can be a relaxing way to transition from the busyness of the day to a state of calm before sleep. Choose reading material that is light and enjoyable, such as fiction, poetry, or inspirational literature, and avoid stimulating or suspenseful content that may interfere with sleep.

8. Listen to Soothing Music or White Noise: Listening to soothing music or white noise can help drown out background noise and create a peaceful sleep environment. Choose calming instrumental music, nature sounds, or white noise recordings to promote relaxation and mask disruptive sounds.

9. Practice Gratitude or Journaling: Take a few moments before bed to reflect on the positive aspects of your day and express gratitude for the things you're thankful for. Alternatively, keep a gratitude journal and write down three things you're grateful for each night. Cultivating a mindset of gratitude can promote feelings of contentment and relaxation before sleep.

10. Create a Comfortable Sleep Environment: Ensure that your bedroom is conducive to sleep by creating a comfortable and relaxing sleep environment. Keep the room cool, dark, and quiet, and invest in a supportive mattress, pillows, and bedding to enhance comfort during sleep.

11. Limit Stimulants and Heavy Meals: Avoid consuming caffeine, nicotine, and heavy or spicy meals close to bedtime, as they can interfere with sleep onset and disrupt sleep quality. Opt for light, easily digestible snacks if you need a bedtime snack, and avoid large meals within 2-3 hours of bedtime.

12. Practice Consistency: Consistency is key to the effectiveness of your bedtime routine. Try to follow the same sequence of relaxing activities each night to establish a predictable routine that signals to your body that it's time to wind down and prepare for sleep.

By incorporating these relaxation techniques into your bedtime routine and creating a calming sleep environment, you can promote relaxation, reduce stress, and improve sleep quality, setting the stage for restful and rejuvenating sleep each night. Experiment with different activities and routines to find what works best for you, and prioritize your bedtime routine as an essential part of your overall self-care and wellness routine.

- *Optimizing Your Sleep Environment*

Optimizing your sleep environment is essential for promoting restful and rejuvenating sleep. A conducive sleep environment can help minimize disruptions, reduce stress, and enhance sleep quality. Here's an extensive overview of how to optimize your sleep environment:

1. Create a Comfortable Sleep Surface:

- Invest in a supportive mattress and pillows that promote proper spinal alignment and comfort during sleep. Choose a mattress with the right level of firmness and support for your body type and sleep preferences.
- Replace old or worn-out bedding and pillows regularly to maintain comfort and hygiene.
- Consider using mattress toppers, mattress pads, or memory foam pillows to enhance comfort and alleviate pressure points.

2. Control Room Temperature:

- Keep your bedroom cool and comfortable, ideally between 60-67 degrees Fahrenheit (15-20 degrees Celsius). A cooler room temperature can promote better sleep by facilitating the body's natural temperature regulation and thermoregulatory processes.

- Use fans, air conditioning, or open windows to circulate fresh air and maintain a comfortable sleeping environment.

- Consider using bedding and sleepwear made from breathable, moisture-wicking materials to help regulate body temperature and minimize overheating during sleep.

3. Manage Light Exposure:
- Keep your bedroom dark and minimize exposure to light sources that can disrupt sleep. Use blackout curtains, shades, or blinds to block out external light sources, especially if you live in an urban area or have streetlights outside your window.

- Avoid using electronic devices with bright screens (e.g., smartphones, tablets, computers) in the hour leading up to bedtime, as the blue light emitted from screens can suppress melatonin production and interfere with sleep onset.

- Consider using a dim nightlight or sleep-friendly lighting with warm, soft hues for nighttime navigation if needed.

4. Minimize Noise Disturbances:
   - Reduce noise disruptions in your sleep environment by using earplugs, white noise machines, or soundproofing measures to block out unwanted noise from traffic, neighbors, or household activities.
   - Use soothing sounds such as nature sounds, gentle music, or white noise recordings to mask disruptive noises and create a peaceful sleep environment.

5. Create a Relaxing Atmosphere:
   - Declutter your bedroom and create a peaceful, clutter-free environment that promotes relaxation and restful sleep. Remove unnecessary items from your bedroom, such as electronics, work-related materials, or exercise equipment.

- Use calming scents such as lavender, chamomile, or jasmine to create a relaxing atmosphere in your bedroom. Consider using essential oil diffusers, linen sprays, or scented candles to infuse your sleep environment with soothing aromas.

6. Optimize Bedtime Rituals:
- Establish a calming bedtime routine to signal to your body that it's time to wind down and prepare for sleep. Engage in relaxing activities such as reading, listening to soothing music, or practicing relaxation techniques like deep breathing or meditation.
- Avoid stimulating activities or stressful tasks close to bedtime, as they can interfere with relaxation and sleep onset. Instead, focus on quiet, calming activities that promote relaxation and stress reduction.

7. Consider Sleep Accessories:

- Explore sleep accessories designed to enhance comfort and promote better sleep, such as weighted blankets, sleep masks, or body pillows. These accessories can provide additional support and promote relaxation during sleep.

8. Maintain Cleanliness and Hygiene:
- Keep your bedroom clean, tidy, and free of dust, allergens, and other irritants that can affect sleep quality and respiratory health. Vacuum regularly, wash bedding and curtains frequently, and dust surfaces to maintain cleanliness and hygiene in your sleep environment.

9. Personalize Your Sleep Space:
- Personalize your sleep environment to reflect your preferences and create a sense of comfort and security. Choose bedding, decor, and colors that you find soothing and relaxing, and incorporate personal touches that make your

bedroom a welcoming and inviting space for sleep.

By implementing these strategies and optimizing your sleep environment, you can create a tranquil and restful space that promotes better sleep quality, enhances relaxation, and contributes to overall well-being. Experiment with different techniques to find what works best for you, and prioritize your sleep environment as an essential component of your sleep hygiene routine.

Healthy Eating Habits for Better Sleep

- Foods That Can Aggravate Snoring

Certain foods and dietary habits can exacerbate snoring by promoting congestion, inflammation, or relaxation of the throat muscles and tissues. Avoiding or minimizing the consumption of these foods before bedtime may help reduce snoring symptoms. Here's an extensive overview of foods that can aggravate snoring:

1. **Dairy Products:** Dairy products such as milk, cheese, and yogurt can increase mucus production and lead to nasal congestion, which can worsen snoring symptoms. Avoid consuming dairy products close to bedtime if you are prone to snoring.

2. Fatty Foods: High-fat foods, especially those high in saturated and trans fats, can promote inflammation throughout the body, including the airways. Fried foods, fatty cuts of meat, and processed snacks should be consumed in moderation, particularly in the evening hours.

3. Spicy Foods: Spicy foods, such as hot peppers, curry, and spicy sauces, can irritate the mucous membranes of the throat and nasal passages, leading to congestion and inflammation. Avoid consuming spicy foods close to bedtime if you experience snoring or related symptoms.

4. Alcohol: Alcohol has a relaxing effect on the muscles in the throat and airway, leading to increased relaxation and potential obstruction during sleep. Consuming alcohol before bedtime can exacerbate snoring and may contribute to sleep-disordered breathing, such as obstructive sleep apnea (OSA).

5. **Caffeinated Beverages:** Caffeine is a stimulant that can disrupt sleep patterns and exacerbate snoring symptoms. Avoid consuming caffeinated beverages such as coffee, tea, or energy drinks in the afternoon and evening, as they can interfere with the quality of your sleep and contribute to snoring.

6. **Heavy Meals:** Eating large, heavy meals close to bedtime can increase pressure on the diaphragm and stomach, leading to acid reflux or gastroesophageal reflux disease (GERD). Acid reflux can cause irritation and inflammation in the throat, exacerbating snoring symptoms. Try to eat lighter, smaller meals earlier in the evening to minimize the risk of reflux and snoring.

7. Processed Foods: Processed foods, including packaged snacks, fast food, and convenience meals, often contain high levels of additives, preservatives, and refined carbohydrates, which can contribute to inflammation and exacerbate snoring symptoms. Opt for whole, unprocessed foods whenever possible to support overall health and reduce snoring risk.

8. High-Sugar Foods: Foods high in sugar, such as sugary desserts, candies, and sweetened beverages, can cause blood sugar fluctuations and promote inflammation in the body. Excessive sugar intake may contribute to weight gain and obesity, both of which are risk factors for snoring and sleep apnea.

9. Salty Foods: High-sodium foods can lead to fluid retention and swelling, particularly in the throat and nasal passages, which can contribute to snoring. Minimize your intake of salty foods such as processed snacks, canned soups, and salty condiments to reduce the risk of snoring-related congestion and inflammation.

10. Acidic Foods: Acidic foods and beverages, such as citrus fruits, tomatoes, and citrus juices, can increase acidity in the stomach and trigger acid reflux, which may worsen snoring symptoms. Limit your consumption of acidic foods in the evening to minimize the risk of reflux and throat irritation.

By being mindful of your dietary choices and avoiding foods that can aggravate snoring, you can reduce the frequency and severity of snoring episodes, improve sleep quality, and support overall respiratory health. Incorporate a balanced and wholesome diet rich in fruits, vegetables, whole grains, lean proteins, and healthy fats to promote better sleep and overall well-being.

- Snoring-Friendly Diet Tips

Adopting a snoring-friendly diet can help reduce snoring by promoting nasal and throat health, supporting optimal weight management, and minimizing inflammation in the airways. Here are some diet tips to help reduce snoring:

1. Stay Hydrated: Drink plenty of water throughout the day to keep mucous membranes in the throat and nasal passages moist and lubricated. Adequate hydration can help reduce congestion and alleviate snoring symptoms.

2. Include Anti-Inflammatory Foods: Incorporate foods that have anti-inflammatory properties into your diet, such as fruits, vegetables, whole grains, nuts, seeds, and fatty fish. These foods contain antioxidants and nutrients that help reduce inflammation in the body, including the airways.

3. Eat Lean Proteins: Choose lean sources of protein, such as poultry, fish, beans, lentils, tofu, and low-fat dairy products, over fatty or processed meats. Lean proteins provide essential nutrients without excess saturated fat, which can contribute to inflammation and snoring.

4. Consume Omega-3 Fatty Acids: Include foods rich in omega-3 fatty acids, such as salmon, mackerel, sardines, flaxseeds, chia seeds, and walnuts, in your diet. Omega-3 fatty acids have anti-inflammatory properties and may help reduce inflammation in the airways, potentially reducing snoring.

5. Limit Salt Intake: Reduce your intake of high-sodium foods and processed snacks, as excess salt can lead to fluid retention and swelling, particularly in the throat and nasal passages. Opt for low-sodium options and use herbs, spices, and other flavorings to season your meals instead of salt.

6. Avoid Heavy Meals Before Bed: Eat lighter meals in the evening and avoid heavy or large meals close to bedtime, as they can increase pressure on the diaphragm and stomach, leading to acid reflux or GERD. Acid reflux can irritate the throat and exacerbate snoring symptoms.

7. Limit Alcohol Consumption: Limit your intake of alcohol, especially in the hours leading up to bedtime. Alcohol has a relaxing effect on the muscles in the throat and airway, which can contribute to increased relaxation and potential obstruction during sleep, leading to snoring.

8. Minimize Caffeine and Stimulants: Reduce your consumption of caffeine-containing beverages such as coffee, tea, and soda, particularly in the afternoon and evening. Caffeine is a stimulant that can interfere with sleep quality and exacerbate snoring symptoms.

9. Eat Smaller, More Frequent Meals: Opt for smaller, more frequent meals throughout the day to maintain stable blood sugar levels and prevent overeating. Spikes and crashes in blood sugar can disrupt sleep patterns and contribute to snoring.

10. Practice Portion Control: Be mindful of portion sizes and avoid overeating, especially at dinner. Eating large meals can increase pressure on the diaphragm and stomach, leading to acid reflux and potentially worsening snoring symptoms.

11. Chew Thoroughly: Chew your food slowly and thoroughly to aid digestion and prevent swallowing excess air, which can contribute to bloating and gas. Swallowing air can also lead to belching, which may disrupt sleep and exacerbate snoring.

12. Consult with a Dietitian: If you have specific dietary concerns or medical conditions that may contribute to snoring, consider consulting with a registered dietitian or nutritionist for personalized dietary recommendations and guidance.

By incorporating these snoring-friendly diet tips into your daily routine, you can support respiratory health, promote optimal weight management, and reduce the frequency and severity of snoring episodes. Combined with other lifestyle modifications and interventions, such as maintaining a healthy weight, practicing good sleep hygiene, and addressing underlying medical conditions, a balanced diet can contribute to better sleep quality and overall well-being.

- The Role of Weight Management

Weight management plays a significant role in the prevention and management of snoring, particularly in individuals who are overweight or obese. Excess weight, especially around the neck and throat area, can contribute to airway obstruction, leading to snoring and sleep-disordered breathing conditions such as obstructive sleep apnea (OSA). Here's an extensive overview of the role of weight management in addressing snoring:

1. Reduction of Excess Fat Deposits: Carrying excess weight, particularly around the neck and throat, can lead to the accumulation of fatty tissues that may narrow the airway and obstruct airflow during sleep. Losing weight can reduce the size of these fat deposits, opening up the airway and reducing the likelihood of snoring.

2. Improvement in Airway Patency: Weight loss can lead to improvements in airway patency and muscle tone in the throat and neck region. As excess weight is lost, there is less pressure on the airway, allowing for easier breathing and reducing the risk of airway collapse or obstruction during sleep.

3. Reduction in Neck Circumference: Excess neck circumference, often associated with obesity, is a significant risk factor for snoring and sleep apnea. By reducing overall body weight, particularly abdominal and neck fat, individuals can experience a decrease in neck circumference, which can improve airflow and reduce snoring severity.

4. Decrease in Fat Deposition in the Tongue and Soft Palate: Weight loss can lead to a reduction in fat deposition in the soft tissues of the throat, tongue, and soft palate, which may contribute to airway obstruction and snoring. By reducing overall body fat percentage, individuals may experience less tissue collapse and obstruction during sleep, leading to improved breathing and reduced snoring.

5. Improvement in Sleep Quality: Losing weight can lead to improvements in sleep quality and architecture, resulting in fewer disruptions and awakenings during the night. Better sleep quality can reduce daytime sleepiness, fatigue, and irritability, all of which may be exacerbated by snoring-related sleep disturbances.

6. Reduction in Risk of Sleep Apnea: Obesity is a significant risk factor for obstructive sleep apnea (OSA), a serious sleep disorder characterized by repetitive episodes of complete or partial upper airway obstruction during sleep. Weight loss can significantly reduce the severity of OSA and may even lead to complete resolution of symptoms in some cases.

7. **Enhancement of Treatment Efficacy:** For individuals with snoring or sleep apnea who require treatment with continuous positive airway pressure (CPAP) therapy or oral appliances, weight loss can improve treatment efficacy and compliance. With less excess weight pressing on the airway, CPAP therapy may be more effective in maintaining airway patency and reducing snoring and apnea events.

8. **Lifestyle Modification:** Weight management often involves adopting healthier lifestyle habits, such as regular exercise, balanced nutrition, and stress management, which can have additional

benefits for overall health and well-being. These lifestyle changes can complement other snoring treatment strategies and contribute to long-term success in managing snoring and related sleep disorders.

In summary, weight management plays a crucial role in addressing snoring and sleep-disordered breathing by reducing excess fat deposition, improving airway patency, and enhancing sleep quality. For individuals who are overweight or obese, incorporating healthy lifestyle habits, such as regular physical activity and nutritious eating, can support weight loss efforts and reduce the severity of snoring symptoms. Additionally, weight management interventions may complement other snoring treatments and improve overall outcomes for individuals with snoring-related sleep disorders.

Avoiding Alcohol and Sedatives

- Understanding the Effects of Alcohol on Sleep

Alcohol can have significant effects on sleep quality and architecture, impacting various stages of the sleep cycle and contributing to sleep disturbances. While alcohol may initially have sedative effects and promote relaxation, its overall impact on sleep can be detrimental. Here's an extensive overview of the effects of alcohol on sleep:

1. Impact on Sleep Onset: Alcohol has sedative properties that can promote sleep onset, making it easier to fall asleep initially. It can also reduce the time it takes to fall asleep, known as sleep latency. However, this initial sedative effect may be short-lived and followed by disruptions in later stages of sleep.

2. Disruption of Sleep Architecture: Alcohol can disrupt the normal progression of sleep stages, including rapid eye movement (REM) sleep and non-rapid eye movement (NREM) sleep. While alcohol may increase the amount of deep NREM sleep in the first half of the night, it tends to suppress REM sleep, resulting in an imbalance in sleep architecture.

3. Fragmented Sleep: Consumption of alcohol before bedtime can lead to fragmented or disrupted sleep, characterized by frequent awakenings throughout the night. These awakenings may occur as the sedative effects of alcohol wear off, leading to periods of wakefulness and difficulty maintaining continuous sleep.

4. Increased Sleep Apnea Risk: Alcohol relaxes the muscles in the throat and airway, leading to increased collapsibility of the upper airway during sleep. This relaxation can exacerbate snoring and may contribute to the development or worsening of sleep-disordered breathing conditions such as obstructive sleep apnea (OSA).

5. Worsening of Sleep-Related Breathing Disorders: For individuals with existing sleep-related breathing disorders such as sleep apnea, alcohol consumption can worsen symptoms and increase the frequency and severity of breathing pauses and oxygen desaturations during sleep. This can lead to daytime sleepiness, fatigue, and other negative health consequences.

6. Decreased Sleep Quality: Despite its initial sedative effects, alcohol consumption can lead to decreased overall sleep quality and feelings of restfulness upon waking. Sleep that is disrupted or fragmented by alcohol may not be as restorative as uninterrupted sleep, leading to daytime drowsiness and impaired cognitive function.

7. Increased Risk of Insomnia: Regular alcohol consumption, particularly in the evening or close to bedtime, can disrupt sleep patterns and contribute to the development of insomnia. Chronic alcohol use can lead to dependence and withdrawal symptoms that further disrupt sleep and perpetuate the cycle of insomnia.

8. Impact on Sleep-Related Hormones: Alcohol can disrupt the normal secretion of hormones involved in sleep regulation, such as melatonin and cortisol. Disruptions in these hormonal rhythms can affect the timing and quality of sleep and may contribute to sleep disturbances and circadian rhythm disorders.

9. Interference with REM Rebound: REM rebound refers to an increase in the duration and intensity of REM sleep following a period of REM suppression. While alcohol initially suppresses REM sleep, discontinuation of alcohol use can lead to rebound effects, including more intense and vivid dreams, which may disrupt sleep continuity.

10. Impaired Next-Day Functioning: Poor sleep quality due to alcohol consumption can impair cognitive function, memory consolidation, and daytime alertness. Individuals may experience increased daytime sleepiness, fatigue, mood disturbances, and impaired performance on cognitive tasks following a night of alcohol-induced sleep disturbances.

In summary, while alcohol may have sedative effects and promote sleep onset, its overall impact on sleep quality and architecture can be detrimental. Regular or excessive alcohol consumption before bedtime can disrupt sleep patterns, exacerbate sleep-related breathing disorders, and impair next-day functioning. Limiting alcohol intake, particularly in the hours leading up to bedtime, can help promote better sleep quality and overall well-being.

- *Identifying Sedatives That Can Worsen Snoring*

Several sedatives and medications have the potential to worsen snoring by relaxing the muscles in the throat and airway, leading to increased airway collapse and obstruction during sleep. These medications can exacerbate snoring symptoms and contribute to sleep-disordered breathing conditions such as obstructive sleep apnea (OSA). Here are some common sedatives and medications that may worsen snoring:

1. **Alcohol:** While not a medication in the traditional sense, alcohol has sedative properties that can relax the muscles in the throat and airway, leading to increased collapsibility of the upper airway during sleep. Alcohol consumption before bedtime can exacerbate snoring and may contribute to the development or worsening of sleep-related breathing disorders such as OSA.

2. **Benzodiazepines:** Benzodiazepines are a class of sedative medications commonly used to treat anxiety, insomnia, and other conditions. Drugs such as diazepam (Valium), lorazepam (Ativan), and clonazepam (Klonopin) can cause muscle relaxation, including the muscles in the throat and airway, potentially increasing the risk of airway collapse and snoring.

3. Non-Benzodiazepine Sedative-Hypnotics: Non-benzodiazepine sedative-hypnotic medications, also known as "Z-drugs," are commonly prescribed for the treatment of insomnia. Drugs such as zolpidem (Ambien), eszopiclone (Lunesta), and zaleplon (Sonata) can have muscle relaxant effects that may contribute to airway collapse and exacerbate snoring.

4. Muscle Relaxants: Muscle relaxant medications are commonly used to treat muscle spasms, tension, and pain. Drugs such as cyclobenzaprine (Flexeril), baclofen (Lioresal), and methocarbamol (Robaxin) can induce muscle relaxation throughout the body, including the muscles in the throat and airway, potentially worsening snoring symptoms.

5. Antihistamines: Some over-the-counter and prescription antihistamine medications, commonly used to treat allergies, colds, and insomnia, can have sedating effects that may contribute to snoring. Antihistamines such as diphenhydramine (Benadryl), doxylamine (Unisom), and cetirizine (Zyrtec) can cause muscle relaxation and increase the risk of airway collapse during sleep.

6. **Opioids:** Opioid medications, commonly prescribed for pain management, can have respiratory depressant effects that may exacerbate snoring and increase the risk of sleep-related breathing disorders. Drugs such as oxycodone (OxyContin), hydrocodone (Vicodin), and morphine can depress respiratory drive and increase the likelihood of airway collapse during sleep.

7. **Antidepressants:** Some antidepressant medications, particularly those with sedative effects, may relax

the muscles in the throat and airway and worsen snoring symptoms. Drugs such as tricyclic antidepressants (e.g., amitriptyline, nortriptyline) and certain selective serotonin reuptake inhibitors (SSRIs) and serotonin-norepinephrine reuptake inhibitors (SNRIs) may have these effects.

It's essential to be aware of the potential side effects of sedatives and medications and their impact on snoring and sleep quality. If you experience worsening snoring or sleep disturbances while taking any medication, consult with your healthcare provider for further evaluation and management. They may recommend adjusting your medication regimen or exploring alternative treatments to address your symptoms effectively while minimizing the risk of snoring-related complications.

- Strategies for Reducing Dependency on Sleep Aids

Reducing dependency on sleep aids involves adopting healthy sleep habits and lifestyle changes to improve sleep quality naturally. Here are some strategies to help reduce reliance on sleep aids:

1. Establish a Consistent Sleep Schedule: Go to bed and wake up at the same time every day, even on weekends. Consistency helps regulate your body's internal clock and promotes better sleep quality.

2. Create a Relaxing Bedtime Routine: Develop a calming bedtime routine to signal to your body that it's time to wind down. Engage in activities such as reading, taking a warm bath, or practicing relaxation techniques like deep breathing or meditation.

3. Optimize Your Sleep Environment: Create a comfortable and conducive sleep environment that promotes relaxation and restorative sleep. Keep your bedroom cool, dark, and quiet, and invest in a comfortable mattress and pillows.

4. Limit Stimulants and Alcohol: Reduce or eliminate consumption of stimulants such as caffeine and nicotine, especially in the afternoon and evening. Avoid alcohol before bedtime, as it can disrupt sleep patterns and worsen snoring.

5. Exercise Regularly: Engage in regular physical activity during the day, but avoid vigorous exercise close to bedtime. Exercise promotes better sleep quality and can help reduce stress and anxiety.

6. Practice Stress Management: Manage stress and anxiety through relaxation techniques such as yoga, mindfulness meditation, or progressive muscle relaxation. Find healthy coping mechanisms to deal with stressors in your life.

7. Limit Screen Time Before Bed: Avoid electronic devices such as smartphones, tablets, and computers before bedtime, as the blue light emitted from screens can interfere with melatonin production and disrupt sleep.

8. Watch Your Diet: Be mindful of your eating habits, especially in the evening. Avoid heavy or spicy meals close to bedtime, and limit consumption of caffeine and sugary foods that can interfere with sleep.

9. Consider Cognitive Behavioral Therapy for Insomnia (CBT-I): CBT-I is a structured program that addresses the underlying causes of insomnia and teaches strategies to improve sleep quality without medication. It focuses on changing behaviors and thought patterns that contribute to sleep difficulties.

10. Gradually Reduce Sleep Aid Use: If you're currently using sleep aids, talk to your healthcare provider about gradually tapering off them. Abruptly stopping sleep aids can lead to rebound insomnia or withdrawal symptoms. Your healthcare provider can provide guidance on safe tapering methods and alternative strategies for improving sleep.

11. Seek Professional Help: If you're struggling to reduce dependency on sleep aids or experiencing chronic sleep difficulties, seek help from a healthcare provider or sleep specialist. They can evaluate your sleep patterns, identify underlying sleep disorders or contributing factors, and recommend personalized treatment options.

By implementing these strategies and making healthy lifestyle changes, you can reduce dependency on sleep aids and improve your overall sleep quality naturally. It may take time and persistence, but with consistent effort, you can achieve better sleep without relying on medication.

Practical Techniques

- Positional Therapy

Positional therapy is a non-invasive approach aimed at reducing snoring and obstructive sleep apnea (OSA) by altering sleep position. It involves encouraging individuals to sleep in positions that minimize airway obstruction and promote optimal breathing throughout the night. For many people, snoring and sleep apnea are more pronounced when sleeping on their back, a position that can lead to the tongue and soft tissues of the throat collapsing backward and obstructing the airway.

By encouraging individuals to sleep on their side or in a slightly elevated position, positional therapy aims to prevent the tongue and soft palate from collapsing into the airway, thus reducing the severity of snoring and sleep apnea events. Sleeping on one's side can help keep the airway open and free of obstruction, allowing for smoother airflow and improved breathing during sleep.

There are several strategies and devices available to facilitate positional therapy, including specialized pillows, positional alarms, and wearable devices designed to promote side sleeping. These devices work by either providing physical support to maintain side sleeping position or alerting individuals when they shift onto their back during sleep, prompting them to change positions.

Positional therapy may be particularly beneficial for individuals with mild to moderate sleep apnea who primarily experience breathing disruptions when sleeping on their back. However, it may not be effective for everyone, especially those with severe sleep apnea or underlying anatomical factors that contribute to airway obstruction regardless of sleep position.

In addition to positional therapy, lifestyle modifications such as weight loss, avoidance of alcohol and sedatives before bedtime, and improvement in sleep hygiene practices can also help reduce snoring and sleep apnea symptoms. For individuals with persistent or severe sleep apnea, a comprehensive treatment approach that may include continuous positive airway pressure (CPAP) therapy, oral appliances, or surgery may be recommended in conjunction with positional therapy for optimal management of the condition.

- *Sleeping Positions That Reduce Snoring*
Several sleeping positions may help reduce snoring by minimizing airway obstruction and promoting optimal

breathing during sleep. Here are some sleeping positions that may be effective in reducing snoring:

1. Side Sleeping: Sleeping on your side, particularly the left side, can help keep the airway open and prevent the tongue and soft tissues of the throat from collapsing backward. This position can promote smoother airflow and reduce the severity of snoring and sleep apnea events.

2. Fetal Position: Curling up on your side with your knees drawn up toward your chest, resembling the fetal position, can help reduce snoring by opening up the airway and preventing the tongue from falling back into the throat. This position may be particularly beneficial for individuals who snore when sleeping on their back.

3. Semi-Fetal Position: Sleeping on your side with your upper body slightly tilted forward and your knees bent can create a semi-fetal position that promotes optimal airway alignment and reduces the risk of snoring. Placing a pillow between your knees can enhance comfort and support in this position.

4. Elevated Head Position: Sleeping with your head elevated on pillows or an adjustable bed can help reduce snoring by preventing the tongue and soft palate from collapsing backward and obstructing the airway. Elevating the head and upper body can promote better breathing and reduce the severity of snoring and sleep apnea events.

5. Modified Prone Position: While sleeping on your stomach (prone position) may not be recommended for everyone, some individuals find relief from snoring by adopting a modified prone position with their head turned to one side. This position may help keep the airway open and reduce the risk of snoring, although it may not be suitable for everyone and can potentially strain the neck and spine.

6. Side-to-Side Rotation: Alternating between sleeping on your right side and left side throughout the night can prevent prolonged pressure on one side of the body and reduce the risk of snoring associated with sleeping exclusively on one side. This rotational approach can help maintain optimal airway alignment and promote restful sleep.

7. Pillow Support: Using pillows strategically to support your head, neck, and body can help maintain proper spinal alignment and promote optimal breathing during sleep. Experiment with different pillow configurations to find what works best for you in reducing snoring and enhancing sleep quality.

While these sleeping positions may help reduce snoring for some individuals, it's essential to find the position that feels most comfortable and natural for you. Additionally, incorporating lifestyle modifications such as weight management, avoidance of alcohol and sedatives before bedtime, and improvement in sleep hygiene practices can further support efforts to reduce snoring and improve overall sleep quality. If snoring persists despite trying different sleeping positions and lifestyle changes, it's important to consult with a healthcare provider for further evaluation and management.

- Using Pillows and Wedges for Positional Therapy

Pillows and wedges are commonly used in positional therapy to promote side sleeping and elevate the head and upper body, reducing the risk of snoring and obstructive sleep apnea (OSA). These supportive devices can help maintain optimal airway alignment and minimize airway obstruction during sleep. Here's how pillows and wedges can be used for positional therapy:

1. Side-Sleeping Pillows: Specialized pillows designed to encourage side sleeping can help keep the airway open and prevent the tongue and soft tissues of the throat from collapsing backward. These pillows often feature a contoured shape that provides support for the head, neck, and shoulders while promoting a comfortable side-sleeping position. Some side-sleeping pillows may also have a raised edge or armrest to prevent rolling onto the back during sleep.

2. Body Pillows: Body pillows are long, cylindrical pillows that can be hugged or placed between the knees to provide support and alignment for the entire body. By placing a body pillow alongside the torso while sleeping on one's side, individuals can maintain a stable side-sleeping position and reduce the risk of rolling onto the back. Body pillows can also help alleviate pressure points and improve overall comfort during sleep.

3. Wedge Pillows: Wedge pillows are triangular-shaped pillows that can be placed under the upper body to elevate the head and upper torso. By elevating the head and neck, wedge pillows help reduce snoring by preventing the tongue and soft palate from collapsing backward and obstructing the airway. Wedge pillows are available in various sizes and degrees of incline to accommodate individual comfort preferences and sleep needs.

4. Adjustable Beds: Adjustable beds allow for customized positioning of the head and upper body, providing a comfortable and supportive sleep surface for individuals with snoring or sleep apnea. By raising the head and upper body, adjustable beds can help reduce snoring and promote optimal breathing during sleep. Some adjustable beds also offer features such as massage functions and programmable presets for added comfort and convenience.

5. Inflatable Positioning Devices: Inflatable positional therapy devices, such as inflatable pillows or wedges, provide adjustable support for side sleeping and head elevation. These devices can be inflated or deflated to achieve the desired level of support and comfort, making them suitable for travel or use in different sleeping environments.

When using pillows and wedges for positional therapy, it's essential to find the right combination of support and comfort that works best for you. Experiment with different pillow configurations and sleeping positions to determine what helps reduce snoring and improve sleep quality. Additionally, incorporating lifestyle modifications such as weight management, avoidance of alcohol and sedatives before bedtime, and improvement in sleep hygiene practices can further enhance the effectiveness of positional therapy for snoring and sleep apnea. If snoring persists despite using pillows and wedges or if you experience other symptoms of sleep-disordered breathing, consult with a healthcare provider for further evaluation and management.

- Training Yourself to Sleep in a Preferred Position

Training yourself to sleep in a preferred position, such as on your side, can be achieved through a combination of behavioral techniques and supportive aids. Here's how you can train yourself to sleep in a preferred position:

1. **Set Intentions:** Before bedtime, set a clear intention to sleep in your preferred position, such as on your side. Visualize yourself comfortably sleeping in that position and affirm your commitment to maintaining it throughout the night.

2. **Use Pillows and Supports:** Place pillows strategically to support your body and encourage side sleeping. A body pillow or a specially designed side-sleeping pillow can provide support and help prevent rolling onto your back. Place a pillow between your knees to alleviate pressure and maintain alignment.

3. **Start Gradually:** If you're accustomed to sleeping in a different position, such as on your back or stomach, transition gradually to your preferred position. Begin by spending a portion of the night in your desired position and gradually increase the duration over time.

4. Practice Relaxation Techniques: Engage in relaxation techniques such as deep breathing, progressive muscle relaxation, or guided imagery before bedtime to promote a calm and restful state of mind. Relaxing your body and mind can make it easier to fall asleep and maintain your preferred sleeping position.

5. Use Positional Alarms: Positional alarms or vibration devices can provide feedback when you shift out of your preferred sleeping position. Place the alarm on your back or chest, and it will alert you with a gentle vibration if you start to roll onto your back. Over time, this feedback can help train your body to stay in your preferred position.

6. Create a Comfortable Sleep Environment: Make your sleep environment conducive to side sleeping by using a supportive mattress and pillows. Ensure that your bedroom is cool, dark, and quiet to promote relaxation and restorative sleep in your preferred position.

7. Be Patient and Persistent: Training yourself to sleep in a preferred position may take time and persistence. Be patient with yourself and acknowledge that it's normal to experience some resistance or discomfort initially. With consistent practice and reinforcement, your body will gradually adapt to your preferred sleeping position.

8. Seek Professional Guidance: If you're struggling to maintain your preferred sleeping position or experiencing persistent sleep difficulties, consider seeking guidance from a healthcare provider or sleep specialist. They can provide personalized recommendations and strategies to address your specific sleep needs and preferences.

By incorporating these techniques and supports into your bedtime routine, you can train yourself to sleep comfortably in your preferred position, such as on your side, and promote better sleep quality and overall well-being. Remember to be patient and persistent, as it may take time for your body to adjust to the new sleeping habit.

- Nasal Congestion Relief

- Identifying Nasal Congestion Triggers

Identifying nasal congestion triggers involves recognizing factors that may exacerbate congestion and contribute to nasal obstruction. By identifying and avoiding these triggers, individuals with nasal congestion can better manage their symptoms and reduce discomfort. Here are common nasal congestion triggers to consider:

1. **Allergens:** Allergens such as pollen, dust mites, pet dander, mold, and certain foods can trigger allergic reactions and nasal congestion in susceptible individuals. Identifying specific allergens through allergy testing and taking steps to minimize exposure, such as using air purifiers, washing bedding frequently, and keeping pets out of the bedroom, can help reduce congestion.

2. **Environmental Irritants:** Exposure to environmental irritants such as cigarette smoke, air pollution, strong odors, and chemicals can irritate the nasal passages and lead to congestion. Minimizing exposure to these irritants by avoiding smoking, using air filters, and improving indoor air quality can help alleviate congestion symptoms.

3. **Weather Changes:** Changes in weather, particularly cold temperatures and low humidity levels, can exacerbate

nasal congestion by drying out the nasal passages and causing inflammation. Using humidifiers to add moisture to the air, staying hydrated, and wearing appropriate clothing to protect against cold weather can help prevent congestion during weather changes.

4. Respiratory Infections: Viral infections such as the common cold, flu, sinusitis, and respiratory syncytial virus (RSV) can cause inflammation of the nasal passages and lead to congestion. Practicing good hygiene, such as frequent handwashing and avoiding close contact with sick individuals, can help reduce the risk of respiratory infections and congestion.

5. Sinus Irritants: Irritants that affect the sinuses, such as dry air, pollution, allergens, and changes in air pressure (e.g., during air travel or scuba diving), can trigger sinus congestion. Taking precautions such as using nasal saline sprays, staying hydrated, and using nasal decongestants as needed can help alleviate sinus-related congestion.

6. **Certain Medications:** Some medications, including decongestants, antihistamines, nasal steroids, and blood pressure medications, can cause nasal congestion as a side effect. If nasal congestion occurs after starting a new medication, consulting with a healthcare provider about alternative treatments or adjusting the dosage may be necessary.

7. **Hormonal Changes:** Hormonal changes, such as those associated with pregnancy, menstruation, menopause, or thyroid disorders, can affect nasal congestion. Managing underlying hormonal imbalances and discussing symptom management strategies with a healthcare provider can help alleviate congestion related to hormonal changes.

8. Food and Beverage Triggers: Certain foods and beverages, such as spicy foods, alcoholic beverages, dairy products, and caffeine, can exacerbate nasal congestion in some individuals. Identifying and avoiding specific triggers can help reduce congestion symptoms.

9. Structural Abnormalities: Structural abnormalities of the nose, such as deviated septum, nasal polyps, or enlarged turbinates, can contribute to chronic nasal congestion. Seeking evaluation and treatment from an otolaryngologist (ear, nose, and throat specialist) can help address underlying structural issues and alleviate congestion symptoms.

By identifying and addressing nasal congestion triggers, individuals can take proactive steps to manage their symptoms and improve nasal health. Keeping a journal to track symptoms and potential triggers can be helpful in identifying patterns and determining effective management strategies. Additionally, consulting with a healthcare provider or allergist can provide personalized guidance and treatment options for managing nasal congestion.

- Home Remedies for Clearing Nasal Passages

Clearing nasal passages at home can provide relief from congestion caused by allergies, colds, sinus infections, or other respiratory conditions. Here are some effective home remedies for clearing nasal passages:

1. Saline Nasal Irrigation: Saline nasal irrigation, also known as nasal saline wash or nasal douche, involves flushing the nasal passages with a saline solution to remove mucus, allergens, and irritants. Use a squeeze bottle, neti pot, or saline nasal spray to irrigate each nostril with the saline solution.

Make sure to use sterile or distilled water and follow proper hygiene practices to prevent infections.

2. Steam Inhalation: Inhaling steam can help moisten and loosen mucus, making it easier to clear nasal passages. Boil water in a pot, remove it from the heat, and lean over the pot with a towel draped over your head to trap the steam. Breathe deeply through your nose for several minutes. Adding essential oils such as eucalyptus or peppermint to the water can enhance the decongestant effects.

3. Warm Compress: Applying a warm compress over the sinuses can help reduce congestion and sinus pressure. Soak a clean washcloth in warm water, wring out excess water, and place it over the nose and sinuses for several minutes. Reapply as needed to alleviate discomfort and promote nasal drainage.

4. Hydration: Drinking plenty of fluids, such as water, herbal teas, and clear broths, can help thin mucus and promote nasal drainage. Staying hydrated helps maintain moisture in the nasal passages and reduces congestion.

5. Humidifier: Using a humidifier in your bedroom can add moisture to the air and help relieve nasal congestion caused by dry indoor air. Keep the humidifier clean to prevent the growth of mold and bacteria, and use distilled or demineralized water to avoid mineral buildup.

6. Nasal Strips: Over-the-counter nasal strips can help open nasal passages and improve airflow, reducing congestion and snoring. Apply a nasal strip across the bridge of the nose before bedtime to help reduce nighttime congestion and improve sleep quality.

7. Elevation: Elevating the head of your bed or using extra pillows to elevate your head and upper body can help reduce nasal congestion by preventing mucus from pooling in the sinuses. Sleeping in a slightly upright position can promote nasal drainage and alleviate discomfort.

8. Spicy Foods: Consuming spicy foods containing ingredients such as chili peppers, horseradish, and mustard can help temporarily relieve nasal congestion by stimulating mucus production and promoting nasal drainage. Incorporate spicy foods into your meals or try adding hot sauce or wasabi to your dishes.

9. Nasal Decongestants: Over-the-counter nasal decongestant sprays or drops can provide temporary relief from nasal congestion by shrinking swollen nasal tissues and reducing inflammation. However, prolonged use of nasal decongestants can lead to rebound congestion, so use them sparingly and follow package instructions carefully.

10. **Avoiding Irritants:** Minimize exposure to irritants such as cigarette smoke, air pollution, strong odors, and allergens that can worsen nasal congestion. Keep windows closed during high pollen seasons, use air purifiers to filter indoor air, and avoid smoking or exposure to secondhand smoke.

By incorporating these home remedies into your daily routine, you can effectively clear nasal passages and alleviate congestion caused by various respiratory conditions. If nasal congestion persists despite home treatment or is accompanied by severe symptoms such as fever, facial pain, or difficulty breathing, consult with a healthcare provider for further evaluation and management.

- Using Nasal Strips and Sprays Effectively

Using nasal strips and sprays effectively can help alleviate nasal congestion and improve breathing. Here's how to use them:

Nasal Strips:

1. Clean and Dry Skin: Before applying a nasal strip, wash your face to remove any dirt, oil, or moisturizers from the skin around your nose. Make sure the skin is completely dry before applying the strip.

2. Positioning: Hold the nasal strip with the tabs in your fingertips. Position the strip so that the center is over the bridge of your nose, just above the flare of your nostrils. The tabs should be on either side of your nostrils.

3. Apply Firmly: Press down on the adhesive sides of the strip to ensure good contact with the skin. Smooth out any wrinkles or air bubbles to create a tight seal. The strip should feel secure but not overly tight or uncomfortable.

4. Breathe Normally: Once the nasal strip is applied, breathe normally through your nose. The strip works by gently lifting and opening the nasal passages, making it easier to breathe and reducing congestion.

5. Remove Carefully: To remove the nasal strip, gently peel it off from both sides. Pulling too quickly or forcefully can cause discomfort or skin irritation. Dispose of the used strip properly.

6. Avoid Overuse: While nasal strips can provide temporary relief from congestion, they are not intended for long-term use. Avoid using nasal strips continuously for extended periods, as prolonged use may lead to skin irritation or dependency on the strips for breathing.

Nasal Sprays:

1. Read Instructions: Before using a nasal spray, carefully read the instructions provided with the product. Pay attention to dosing recommendations, storage instructions, and any precautions or warnings.

2. Shake the Bottle: Shake the nasal spray bottle gently to ensure that the medication is evenly mixed and ready for use. Some nasal sprays may require priming before the first use, so follow the manufacturer's instructions if necessary.

3. Clear Nasal Passages: Blow your nose gently to clear any excess mucus from your nasal passages before using the nasal spray. This allows the medication to reach the nasal tissues more effectively.

4. Tilt Head Forward: Tilt your head slightly forward and insert the nozzle of the nasal spray into one nostril. Keep the bottle upright and aim the nozzle toward the outer wall of the nostril, away from the center of your nose.

5. Administer Spray: Press down on the pump or squeeze the bottle to release a single spray of medication into your nostril. Breathe in gently through your nose as you administer the spray to help the medication reach deeper into your nasal passages.

6. Repeat for Other Nostril: Repeat the process for the other nostril, if instructed by your healthcare provider or the product label. Avoid blowing your nose immediately after using the nasal spray to allow the medication to remain in your nasal passages.

7. Clean Nozzle: After each use, wipe the nozzle of the nasal spray bottle with a clean tissue or cloth to remove any excess medication. Replace the cap securely to prevent contamination or leakage.

8. Follow Usage Guidelines: Use the nasal spray as directed by your healthcare provider or the product label. Avoid using the spray more frequently or for longer than recommended, as overuse can lead to rebound congestion or other side effects.

By using nasal strips and sprays correctly and following recommended guidelines, you can effectively manage nasal congestion and improve breathing comfort. If you have any questions or concerns about using these products, consult with your healthcare provider for personalized advice and recommendations.

- Throat and Tongue Exercises

- Strengthening Exercises for Throat Muscles

Strengthening exercises for throat muscles can help reduce snoring and improve overall airway function by toning and tightening the muscles that support the throat and airway. Here are some effective exercises to strengthen throat muscles:

1. Tongue Presses:

   - Sit upright and stick out your tongue as far as possible.

   - Press the tip of your tongue against the roof of your mouth and hold for 5-10 seconds.

   - Repeat this exercise several times, gradually increasing the duration of each hold.

2. Throat Exercises:

- Open your mouth wide and say "Ahh" as if you were at the doctor's office for a throat examination.
- Hold the "Ahh" position for a few seconds, then relax.
- Repeat this exercise several times to strengthen the muscles at the back of your throat.

3. Gargling:

- Gargling with warm salt water or an antiseptic mouthwash can help strengthen the muscles in the throat and prevent infections.
- Gargle for 30 seconds to 1 minute, then spit out the solution.
- Repeat this exercise several times a day, especially during periods of congestion or throat irritation.

4. Humming:

- Sit or stand comfortably and take a deep breath.

- Exhale slowly while humming the sound "mmm" with your mouth closed.
- Feel the vibrations in your throat and chest as you hum.
- Repeat this exercise for several breaths, focusing on maintaining a steady and smooth hum.

5. Singing:
- Singing exercises the muscles in the throat, palate, and tongue, helping to strengthen and tone them.
- Practice singing scales, vocal warm-up exercises, or your favorite songs to engage the muscles in your throat and improve vocal control.

6. Swallowing Exercises:
- Practice swallowing exercises to strengthen the muscles involved in swallowing and prevent choking or aspiration.
- Take small sips of water and swallow deliberately, focusing on using the muscles in your throat and esophagus.

- Repeat this exercise several times, gradually increasing the volume of water and the intensity of the swallow.

7. Chin Lifts:
  - Sit or stand upright with your shoulders relaxed.
  - Tilt your head back as far as comfortable while keeping your lips closed.
  - Hold this position for a few seconds, then return to the starting position.
  - Repeat this exercise several times to strengthen the muscles in the front of your neck and throat.

8. Jaw Exercises:
  - Open your mouth wide and move your jaw from side to side in a chewing motion.
  - Perform gentle jaw stretches by opening and closing your mouth slowly and deliberately.
  - Repeat these exercises several times to improve jaw mobility and

strengthen the muscles around the throat and neck.

Consistency is key when performing throat strengthening exercises. Aim to incorporate these exercises into your daily routine and gradually increase the intensity and duration over time. If you experience any discomfort or pain while performing these exercises, stop immediately and consult with a healthcare provider or speech therapist for guidance.

- *Tongue Exercises to Prevent Obstruction*

Tongue exercises can help prevent obstruction of the airway by strengthening the muscles in the tongue and surrounding areas, reducing the risk of snoring and obstructive sleep apnea. Here are some effective tongue exercises to incorporate into your daily routine:

1. Tongue Stretch:

- Stick out your tongue as far as possible, reaching towards your chin.
- Hold this position for 5-10 seconds, feeling the stretch in the muscles of your tongue and throat.
- Relax and repeat the stretch several times, gradually increasing the duration of each hold.

2. Tongue Press Against Palate:

- Press the tip of your tongue against the roof of your mouth (palate) with firm pressure.
- Hold this position for 5-10 seconds, then release.
- Repeat the press several times, focusing on engaging the muscles of the tongue and palate.

3. Tongue Push-Ups:

- Press the tip of your tongue against the back of your top front teeth.

- Push upward against the teeth, applying gentle pressure with the tongue.
  - Hold for a few seconds, then relax.
  - Repeat this pushing motion several times to strengthen the muscles of the tongue.

4. Tongue Rolling:
  - Roll your tongue upward and backward towards the roof of your mouth.
  - Hold this rolled position for a few seconds, then unroll the tongue.
  - Repeat the rolling motion several times, focusing on controlling the movement with your tongue muscles.

5. Tongue Side-to-Side Movement:
  - Stick out your tongue and move it from side to side, touching the corners of your mouth.
  - Repeat this side-to-side movement several times, feeling the muscles of your tongue working with each motion.

6. Tongue Resistance Exercise:

- Place the tip of your tongue against the back of your bottom front teeth.
- Push the tongue forward against the teeth, creating resistance with the lower jaw.
- Hold this position for a few seconds, then relax.
- Repeat the resistance exercise several times, focusing on engaging the muscles of the tongue and jaw.

7. Tongue Chewing:

- Mimic the motion of chewing gum with your tongue, pressing it against the roof of your mouth.
- Perform chewing motions with your tongue, moving it up and down and side to side.
- Repeat this tongue chewing exercise for several repetitions, focusing on strengthening the muscles of the tongue and palate.

8. Tongue Scraper:

- Use a tongue scraper to gently clean the surface of your tongue from back to front.

- This helps remove bacteria, debris, and dead cells from the tongue, promoting better oral hygiene and muscle function.

Perform these tongue exercises regularly as part of your daily routine to strengthen the muscles of the tongue and reduce the risk of airway obstruction during sleep. Consistency is key to achieving and maintaining optimal tongue muscle strength and function. If you experience any discomfort or pain while performing these exercises, stop immediately and consult with a healthcare provider for guidance.

- *Incorporating Daily Exercise Routines*

Incorporating daily exercise routines into your lifestyle can improve overall health and well-being, including reducing the risk of snoring and sleep apnea. Here are some tips for integrating exercise into your daily routine:

1. Choose Activities You Enjoy: Select exercises and activities that you genuinely enjoy and look forward to doing. Whether it's walking, jogging, swimming, cycling, dancing, or playing sports, finding activities that you find fun and enjoyable increases the likelihood that you'll stick with them long-term.

2. Set Realistic Goals: Set achievable goals for your exercise routine, such as aiming for a certain number of minutes or steps per day. Start with manageable goals and gradually increase the intensity, duration, and frequency of your workouts as your fitness level improves.

3. Schedule Exercise Time: Treat exercise as an essential part of your daily schedule by blocking out dedicated time for physical activity. Whether it's first thing in the morning, during your lunch break, or in the evening, choose a time that works best for you and stick to it consistently.

4. Incorporate Variety: Incorporate a variety of exercises and activities into your routine to keep things interesting and prevent boredom. Mix cardio exercises with strength training, flexibility exercises, and balance work to target different muscle groups and keep your workouts diverse.

5. Start Small: If you're new to exercise or have been inactive for a while, start with small, manageable steps and gradually increase the intensity and duration of your workouts. Even short bouts of exercise, such as a 10-minute walk, can provide significant health benefits when done regularly.

6. Be Active Throughout the Day: Look for opportunities to be active throughout the day, such as taking the stairs instead of the elevator, walking or biking instead of driving for short trips, or doing household chores and gardening. Every little bit of movement adds up and contributes to your overall activity level.

7. Find Accountability Partners: Exercise with a friend, family member, or workout buddy to help stay motivated and accountable. Having someone to share your fitness journey with can provide encouragement, support, and a sense of camaraderie.

8. Listen to Your Body: Pay attention to how your body feels during and after exercise, and adjust your routine as needed to prevent injury and avoid overexertion. If you experience pain or discomfort, modify your workout or try a different activity that's more suitable for your fitness level and abilities.

9. Prioritize Recovery: Allow time for rest and recovery between workouts to give your body time to repair and rebuild muscle tissue. Incorporate stretching, foam rolling, and relaxation techniques into your routine to promote recovery and reduce muscle soreness.

10. Stay Consistent: Consistency is key to seeing results from your exercise routine. Aim to exercise most days of the week, even if it's just a short duration. Remember that progress takes time, so be patient and stay committed to your fitness goals.

By incorporating daily exercise routines into your lifestyle and making physical activity a priority, you can improve your overall health, reduce the risk of snoring and sleep apnea, and enhance your quality of life. Choose activities that you enjoy, set realistic goals, and stay consistent with your workouts to reap the many benefits of regular exercise.

Devices and Medical Treatments

Devices and medical treatments for snoring and sleep apnea range from non-invasive devices to surgical interventions, depending on the severity and underlying cause of the condition. Continuous positive airway pressure (CPAP) therapy is one of the most common and effective treatments for obstructive sleep apnea (OSA). CPAP therapy involves wearing a mask connected to a machine that delivers a steady stream of air pressure to keep the airway open during sleep, preventing pauses in breathing and reducing snoring. While CPAP therapy is highly effective, some individuals may find it uncomfortable or challenging to use consistently.

For those who are unable to tolerate CPAP therapy or have mild to moderate sleep apnea, oral appliances may be recommended. These devices are custom-fitted by a dentist or orthodontist and are worn in the mouth during sleep to reposition the jaw and tongue, keeping the airway open and reducing snoring and sleep apnea events. Oral appliances are often more comfortable and portable than CPAP machines, making them a popular alternative for some individuals.

Another non-invasive option for treating snoring and sleep apnea is positional therapy. Positional therapy involves using devices such as specialized pillows, positional alarms, or wearable devices to encourage sleeping in positions that minimize airway obstruction and reduce snoring. For individuals whose snoring is primarily positional, such as when sleeping on their back, positional therapy can be an effective treatment option.

In cases where non-invasive treatments are ineffective or not tolerated, surgical interventions may be considered. Surgical options for snoring and sleep apnea may include procedures to remove excess tissue from the throat (uvulopalatopharyngoplasty), reposition the jaw (maxillomandibular advancement), or implant devices to support the soft palate and prevent collapse of the airway during sleep (palatal implants). Surgical treatments are typically reserved for individuals with severe sleep apnea or anatomical abnormalities that contribute to airway obstruction.

In addition to devices and medical treatments, lifestyle modifications such as weight loss, avoidance of alcohol and sedatives before bedtime, and improvement in sleep hygiene practices can also help reduce snoring and improve sleep quality. It's essential for individuals experiencing snoring or sleep apnea to undergo a thorough evaluation by a healthcare provider or sleep specialist to determine the most appropriate treatment approach based on their specific needs and circumstances.

- Oral Appliances for Snoring

Oral appliances are a popular and effective treatment option for snoring and mild to moderate obstructive sleep apnea (OSA). These custom-fitted devices are worn in the mouth during sleep to reposition the jaw and tongue, keeping the airway open and reducing snoring and sleep apnea events. Here's how oral appliances for snoring work and what to expect when using them:

1. **Custom-Fitted Design:** Oral appliances are individually customized to fit the unique shape and size of each person's mouth. They are typically made of acrylic and consist of upper and lower

trays that fit over the teeth and are connected by adjustable hinges or straps.

2. Repositioning the Jaw: Oral appliances work by repositioning the lower jaw (mandible) slightly forward during sleep. This forward positioning helps prevent the tongue and soft tissues of the throat from collapsing backward and obstructing the airway, reducing the severity of snoring and sleep apnea events.

3. Types of Oral Appliances: There are several types of oral appliances available for the treatment of snoring and sleep apnea. Mandibular advancement devices (MADs) are the most common type and work by gradually advancing the lower jaw forward. Tongue-retaining devices (TRDs) hold the tongue in a forward position to prevent it from falling back into the throat.

4. Customization and Adjustment: Oral appliances are custom-fitted by a dentist or orthodontist trained in dental sleep medicine. During the fitting process, detailed impressions and measurements of the mouth are taken to ensure a precise fit. The appliance may be adjusted over time to optimize comfort and effectiveness.

5. Comfort and Convenience: Oral appliances are typically more comfortable and less intrusive than continuous positive airway pressure (CPAP) machines, making them a preferred option for some individuals. They are also portable and easy to travel with, allowing for uninterrupted sleep therapy even while away from home.

6. Regular Follow-Up: After receiving an oral appliance, regular follow-up appointments with the dentist or sleep specialist may be necessary to monitor progress and make any necessary adjustments to the device. Periodic assessments of sleep quality and symptoms may also be conducted to evaluate treatment effectiveness.

7. Potential Side Effects: While oral appliances are generally well-tolerated, some individuals may experience temporary side effects such as jaw discomfort, tooth pain, or excessive salivation during the adjustment period. These side effects usually resolve with time and can often be minimized by adjusting the appliance.

8. Long-Term Use: Oral appliances are typically recommended for long-term use to maintain the benefits of treatment. Regular use of the appliance is essential for optimal effectiveness in reducing snoring and improving sleep quality. It's important to follow the recommendations of the healthcare provider and attend scheduled follow-up appointments to ensure the continued success of treatment.

Overall, oral appliances are a safe, effective, and convenient treatment option for snoring and mild to moderate obstructive sleep apnea. They offer an alternative to CPAP therapy for individuals who are unable to tolerate or prefer not to use a CPAP machine. If you experience snoring or sleep apnea symptoms, consult with a dentist or sleep specialist to determine if an oral appliance may be a suitable treatment option for you.

- How Mandibular Advancement Devices Work

Mandibular advancement devices (MADs) are oral appliances used to treat snoring and obstructive sleep apnea (OSA) by repositioning the lower jaw (mandible) slightly forward during sleep. These devices work by opening the airway and preventing the collapse of soft tissues in the throat, which can lead to airway obstruction and breathing disturbances. Here's how mandibular advancement devices work:

1. Repositioning the Jaw: MADs are designed to hold the lower jaw in a protruded position, slightly advancing it forward relative to the upper jaw (maxilla). By repositioning the jaw in this manner, MADs help enlarge the upper airway and create more space for airflow during sleep.

2. Tension on Muscles and Tissues: When the lower jaw is advanced forward, it places tension on the muscles and soft tissues at the back of the throat. This tension helps prevent the tongue and soft palate from collapsing backward and obstructing the airway, reducing the severity of snoring and sleep apnea events.

3. Maintaining Airway Patency: By maintaining the patency of the upper airway, MADs help prevent episodes of apnea (complete cessation of breathing) or hypopnea (partial reduction in airflow) that occur during sleep in individuals with OSA. By keeping the airway open, MADs promote uninterrupted breathing and improve oxygenation during sleep.

4. Adjustability: Many MADs are adjustable, allowing for customization to fit the individual's mouth and jaw anatomy comfortably. Adjustable MADs typically feature mechanisms such as screws or rods that can be used to incrementally advance or retract the lower jaw to achieve the optimal position for reducing snoring and sleep apnea.

5. Comfort and Compliance: MADs are often more comfortable and less intrusive than continuous positive airway pressure (CPAP) machines, making them a preferred treatment option for some individuals with OSA. The ability to adjust the device to the desired level of advancement helps improve comfort and compliance with treatment.

6. **Effectiveness:** MADs have been shown to be effective in reducing snoring and improving symptoms of mild to moderate obstructive sleep apnea in many individuals. They are particularly beneficial for individuals who are unable to tolerate CPAP therapy or prefer oral appliance therapy as a more convenient and portable treatment option.

7. **Long-Term Use:** MADs are typically recommended for long-term use to maintain the benefits of treatment. Regular use of the device during sleep is essential for optimal effectiveness in reducing snoring and improving sleep quality. Periodic follow-up appointments with a dentist or sleep specialist may be necessary to monitor progress and

make any necessary adjustments to the device.

Overall, mandibular advancement devices are a safe, effective, and convenient treatment option for snoring and obstructive sleep apnea. They offer an alternative to CPAP therapy for individuals who are unable to tolerate or prefer not to use a CPAP machine. If you experience snoring or sleep apnea symptoms, consult with a dentist or sleep specialist to determine if a mandibular advancement device may be a suitable treatment option for you.

- Choosing the Right Oral Appliance

Choosing the right oral appliance for treating snoring or sleep apnea is essential for achieving optimal effectiveness, comfort, and compliance with treatment. Here are some factors to consider when selecting an oral appliance:

1. **Type of Appliance:** There are several types of oral appliances available for the treatment of snoring and sleep apnea, including mandibular advancement devices (MADs) and tongue-retaining devices (TRDs). MADs work by repositioning the lower jaw forward, while TRDs hold the tongue in a forward position to prevent it from collapsing backward into the throat. The type of appliance that is most suitable for you will depend on factors such as your jaw anatomy, the severity of your condition, and your personal preferences.

2. **Customization:** Oral appliances should be custom-fitted by a dentist or orthodontist trained in dental sleep medicine to ensure a precise fit and optimal effectiveness. Customization involves taking detailed impressions and measurements of your mouth to create a device that fits comfortably and

securely. Avoid over-the-counter or one-size-fits-all oral appliances, as they may not provide adequate fit or effectiveness.

3. Comfort: Comfort is a critical factor in selecting an oral appliance, as you will be wearing it during sleep. Look for devices that are made of soft, biocompatible materials and have smooth edges to minimize irritation to the gums, teeth, and soft tissues of the mouth. Adjustable appliances allow for customization of the fit and positioning to maximize comfort.

4. Ease of Use: Choose an oral appliance that is easy to insert, remove, and clean. Devices with simple adjustment mechanisms and user-friendly features make it easier to fine-tune the fit and achieve optimal effectiveness. Consider the ease of maintenance and cleaning, as regular cleaning is essential for prolonging the lifespan of the appliance and ensuring oral hygiene.

5. Effectiveness: The effectiveness of an oral appliance in reducing snoring and improving sleep apnea symptoms is a crucial consideration. Look for devices with evidence-based efficacy and a track record of success in clinical studies. Discuss the expected outcomes and potential side effects with your healthcare provider to ensure that the chosen appliance is appropriate for your specific needs and condition.

6. Durability and Longevity: Choose an oral appliance that is durable and built to withstand nightly use over an extended period. High-quality materials and construction ensure that the device maintains its effectiveness and structural integrity over time. Ask about warranty coverage and replacement policies to ensure peace of mind and investment protection.

7. Compliance: Compliance with oral appliance therapy is essential for achieving optimal treatment outcomes. Select an appliance that you feel comfortable wearing and are motivated to use consistently. Discuss any concerns or preferences with your healthcare provider to ensure that the chosen appliance aligns with your lifestyle and preferences.

8. Cost and Insurance Coverage: Consider the cost of the oral appliance and whether it is covered by your health insurance plan. While some insurance plans may cover a portion of the cost of oral appliances for the treatment of sleep apnea, coverage varies depending on the provider and policy. Discuss payment options and reimbursement with your insurance provider and healthcare provider to understand the financial implications of treatment.

By carefully considering these factors and consulting with a qualified healthcare provider or dentist specializing in dental sleep medicine, you can select the right oral appliance for treating your snoring or sleep apnea effectively and comfortably. Follow-up appointments and ongoing monitoring are essential for ensuring the continued success of treatment and making any necessary adjustments to the appliance.

- Adjusting to Using Oral Appliances

Adjusting to using oral appliances for snoring or sleep apnea treatment can take time and patience as your mouth, jaw, and sleep patterns adapt to the device. Here are some tips to help you adjust to using oral appliances more comfortably and effectively:

1. Start Slowly: Ease into wearing the oral appliance by wearing it for short periods during the day before attempting to use it during sleep. This allows your mouth and jaw muscles to become accustomed to the device gradually.

2. **Follow Instructions:** Follow the instructions provided by your dentist or healthcare provider for wearing and caring for the oral appliance. Proper use and maintenance are essential for optimizing effectiveness and prolonging the lifespan of the device.

3. **Practice Good Oral Hygiene:** Maintain good oral hygiene habits by brushing and flossing your teeth regularly, as well as cleaning the oral appliance according to the manufacturer's recommendations. Clean the appliance thoroughly after each use to remove plaque, bacteria, and debris.

4. **Adjustment Period:** Understand that there may be an adjustment period as your mouth, jaw, and sleep patterns adapt to the oral appliance. It may take

several nights or weeks to become fully accustomed to wearing the device during sleep.

5. Expect Some Discomfort: It's normal to experience some discomfort or minor side effects, such as jaw soreness, tooth discomfort, or excessive salivation, during the initial adjustment period. These symptoms usually subside with time as your body adjusts to the device.

6. Seek Professional Guidance: If you experience persistent discomfort or difficulty adjusting to the oral appliance, consult with your dentist or healthcare provider for guidance. They can make any necessary adjustments to the device or recommend alternative treatment options to improve comfort and effectiveness.

7. Stay Consistent: Consistency is key to achieving optimal results with oral appliance therapy. Wear the device every night as prescribed, even if you don't notice immediate improvements in snoring or sleep apnea symptoms. Over time, consistent use of the appliance can lead to significant reductions in symptoms and improvements in sleep quality.

8. Monitor Progress: Keep track of your progress and any changes in snoring or sleep apnea symptoms after using the oral appliance. If you notice any changes or concerns, discuss them with your healthcare provider to determine the appropriate course of action.

9. Be Patient: Patience is essential when adjusting to using oral appliances for snoring or sleep apnea treatment. Give yourself time to adapt to the device and trust that with patience and persistence, you will experience the benefits of treatment over time.

By following these tips and staying committed to using the oral appliance as prescribed, you can adjust more comfortably and effectively to using the device for snoring or sleep apnea treatment. Remember to communicate any concerns or difficulties with your healthcare provider, who can offer guidance and support throughout the adjustment process.

Continuous Positive Airway Pressure (CPAP) Therapy

- Understanding CPAP Machines and Masks

Understanding CPAP (Continuous Positive Airway Pressure) machines and masks is essential for individuals with obstructive sleep apnea (OSA) who are considering or undergoing CPAP therapy. Here's a closer look at CPAP machines and masks:

1. CPAP Machines: CPAP machines are medical devices that deliver a continuous flow of air at a prescribed pressure to keep the airway open during sleep. The machine consists of a motor, air pump, and humidifier, housed in a compact unit that sits on a bedside table. The air is delivered through a hose connected to the machine and a mask worn over the nose, mouth, or both.

2. **Function:** The primary function of a CPAP machine is to prevent the collapse of the upper airway and maintain sufficient airflow to prevent apneas (pauses in breathing) and hypopneas (shallow breathing) during sleep. By delivering a constant stream of air pressure, CPAP therapy helps alleviate symptoms of OSA, including snoring, daytime sleepiness, and fatigue.

3. **Pressure Settings:** CPAP machines are programmed with adjustable pressure settings that are prescribed by a healthcare provider based on the severity of the individual's sleep apnea. The pressure setting is determined during a sleep study or titration study, where the patient's breathing patterns are monitored to determine the optimal

pressure needed to keep the airway open.

4. Humidification: Many CPAP machines feature integrated humidifiers that add moisture to the air delivered through the mask, reducing dryness and irritation of the nasal passages and throat. Humidification can help improve comfort and compliance with CPAP therapy, especially for individuals who experience dry mouth or nasal congestion.

5. Data Recording: Modern CPAP machines often include built-in data recording capabilities that track usage data, such as hours of use, mask leakages, apnea events, and air pressure settings. This data can be valuable for monitoring treatment adherence, evaluating therapy effectiveness, and making adjustments as needed.

6. Types of Masks: CPAP masks come in various styles and designs to accommodate different preferences and facial structures. The three main types of CPAP masks are nasal masks, nasal pillows, and full-face masks. Nasal masks cover the nose only, nasal pillows insert into the nostrils, and full-face masks cover both the nose and mouth.

7. Mask Fit and Comfort: Proper mask fit and comfort are essential for successful CPAP therapy. A well-fitting mask should create a secure seal against the face without causing discomfort or pressure points. It's important to try different mask styles and sizes to find the one that provides the best fit and comfort for your individual needs.

8. Mask Maintenance: Regular cleaning and maintenance of CPAP masks are essential for ensuring hygiene and prolonging the lifespan of the mask. Most masks can be cleaned with mild soap and water daily and should be replaced periodically as recommended by the manufacturer.

9. **Mask Accessories:** Various accessories are available to enhance mask comfort and usability, such as mask liners, strap pads, and nasal cushions. These accessories can help reduce skin irritation, improve seal integrity, and enhance overall mask comfort during sleep.

10. **Mask Adjustment:** It may take time to adjust to wearing a CPAP mask, especially if you are new to CPAP therapy. Start by wearing the mask for short periods during the day to become accustomed to the sensation. Gradually increase the duration of wear until you can comfortably tolerate wearing the mask throughout the night.

Understanding CPAP machines and masks is crucial for individuals undergoing CPAP therapy for obstructive sleep apnea. By selecting the right equipment, ensuring proper fit and comfort, and adhering to recommended cleaning and maintenance practices, individuals can maximize the effectiveness of CPAP therapy and improve their quality of sleep and overall health. Regular follow-up with a healthcare provider is essential for monitoring progress, adjusting treatment as needed, and addressing any concerns or challenges related to CPAP therapy.

- *Overcoming Common CPAP Challenges*

Overcoming common CPAP (Continuous Positive Airway Pressure) challenges is essential for individuals using CPAP therapy to treat obstructive sleep apnea (OSA) effectively. Here are some common challenges associated with CPAP therapy and strategies for overcoming them:

1. Mask Discomfort: One of the most common challenges with CPAP therapy is mask discomfort, including issues such as skin irritation, pressure sores, or difficulty achieving a proper seal. To overcome mask discomfort:
 - Try different mask styles, sizes, and types to find the one that fits best and feels most comfortable for your individual needs.
 - Adjust the mask straps and positioning to achieve a secure but comfortable fit.
 - Use mask liners, strap pads, or nasal cushions to reduce skin irritation and pressure points.
 - Practice wearing the mask during the day to become accustomed to the sensation before using it during sleep.

2. Dryness or Congestion: CPAP therapy can sometimes cause dryness or congestion in the nasal passages or throat, leading to discomfort or difficulty breathing. To overcome dryness or congestion:

- Use a CPAP machine with an integrated humidifier to add moisture to the air delivered through the mask.

- Adjust the humidity settings on the CPAP machine to the desired level of comfort.

- Use a saline nasal spray or nasal irrigation before bedtime to moisturize the nasal passages and reduce congestion.

- Consider using a heated tube or heated humidification system to enhance humidification and reduce dryness.

3. Mask Leakages: Mask leakages occur when air escapes from the mask, compromising the effectiveness of CPAP therapy and causing disruptions in sleep. To overcome mask leakages:

- Ensure that the mask is fitted properly and creates a secure seal against the face without gaps or leaks.

- Adjust the mask straps and positioning to minimize air leaks and improve seal integrity.

- Replace worn-out mask components, such as cushions, seals, or straps, as needed to maintain a proper fit.

- Practice proper mask hygiene and maintenance to keep the mask clean and free of debris that could interfere with the seal.

4. Claustrophobia or Anxiety: Some individuals may experience feelings of claustrophobia or anxiety when wearing a CPAP mask, especially during the initial adjustment period. To overcome feelings of claustrophobia or anxiety:

- Gradually acclimate to wearing the CPAP mask by starting with short periods of wear during the day and gradually increasing the duration over time.

- Practice relaxation techniques, such as deep breathing, meditation, or visualization, to reduce feelings of anxiety and promote relaxation while wearing the mask.
- Seek support from a healthcare provider, therapist, or support group specializing in sleep disorders for guidance and coping strategies.

5. Difficulty Falling Asleep: Adjusting to CPAP therapy and wearing a mask during sleep can sometimes make it challenging to fall asleep initially. To overcome difficulty falling asleep:
- Establish a relaxing bedtime routine to wind down before sleep, including activities such as reading, listening to calming music, or taking a warm bath.
- Use relaxation techniques, such as progressive muscle relaxation or guided imagery, to promote relaxation and reduce stress or tension before bedtime.
- Experiment with different mask styles, sizes, or positions to find the

most comfortable and conducive to sleep.

- Practice good sleep hygiene habits, such as maintaining a consistent sleep schedule, avoiding caffeine and stimulating activities before bedtime, and creating a comfortable sleep environment.

6. Excessive Noise or Disruption: CPAP machines can sometimes produce noise or vibrations that disrupt sleep or disturb bed partners. To overcome excessive noise or disruption:

- Place the CPAP machine on a stable surface away from the bed to reduce vibrations and noise transmission.

- Use a CPAP machine with a quiet motor and noise-reduction features to minimize disturbances during sleep.

- Consider using a CPAP machine with a ramp feature that gradually increases air pressure over time, allowing for a more gradual adjustment to therapy.

- Use earplugs or white noise machines to mask any residual noise and promote a quieter sleep environment.

7. Feeling Claustrophobic or Confined: For some users, wearing a CPAP mask may feel claustrophobic or confining. To overcome this challenge:

- Gradually increase the duration of mask wear during the day to become more accustomed to the sensation.
- Practice relaxation techniques, such as deep breathing or progressive muscle relaxation, to reduce feelings of anxiety or claustrophobia while wearing the mask.
- Use distraction techniques, such as listening to calming music or engaging in a relaxing activity, to shift your focus away from the mask and promote relaxation.
- Seek support from a healthcare provider or therapist specializing in

sleep disorders for guidance and coping strategies.

By addressing these common challenges and implementing strategies to overcome them, individuals using CPAP therapy can improve comfort, compliance, and effectiveness of treatment for obstructive sleep apnea. It's essential to communicate any concerns or difficulties with your healthcare provider or CPAP equipment provider, who can offer guidance, support, and solutions tailored to your individual needs.

- *CPAP Alternatives and Variations*

Several CPAP alternatives and variations exist for individuals who are unable to tolerate or prefer alternatives to traditional CPAP therapy for treating obstructive sleep apnea (OSA). Here are some CPAP alternatives and variations:

1. **Bi-level Positive Airway Pressure (BiPAP) Therapy:** BiPAP therapy delivers two different levels of air pressure—one for inhalation and a lower pressure for exhalation. This variation may be more comfortable for individuals who have difficulty exhaling against the continuous pressure of traditional CPAP therapy.

2. **Auto-adjusting Positive Airway Pressure (APAP) Therapy:** APAP therapy automatically adjusts the air pressure delivered by the CPAP machine based on the individual's breathing patterns throughout the night. This allows for more personalized and adaptive treatment, optimizing comfort and effectiveness.

3. **Expiratory Positive Airway Pressure (EPAP) Therapy:** EPAP therapy uses disposable adhesive nasal devices that create resistance during

exhalation, helping to keep the airway open. EPAP devices are non-invasive and may be suitable for individuals who prefer nasal treatment options or have difficulty tolerating traditional CPAP masks.

4. **Provent Therapy:** Provent Therapy involves wearing small, disposable nasal patches with one-way valves that create resistance during exhalation, similar to EPAP devices. Provent Therapy is non-invasive and may be suitable for individuals who prefer nasal treatment options or have difficulty tolerating CPAP therapy.

5. **Adaptive Servo-Ventilation (ASV) Therapy:** ASV therapy is designed for individuals with complex sleep apnea or central sleep apnea, which involves interruptions in breathing due to problems with the brain's respiratory control center. ASV therapy delivers varying levels of pressure support to

maintain regular breathing patterns and prevent apneas.

6. Oral Appliance Therapy: Oral appliances are custom-fitted devices worn in the mouth during sleep to reposition the jaw and tongue, keeping the airway open and reducing snoring and sleep apnea events. Oral appliance therapy may be an alternative to CPAP therapy for individuals with mild to moderate OSA or those who prefer oral appliance treatment.

7. Positional Therapy: Positional therapy involves using devices or positional alarms to encourage sleeping in positions that minimize airway obstruction and reduce snoring. Positional therapy may be beneficial for individuals whose sleep apnea is primarily positional, such as when sleeping on their back.

8. Surgical Interventions: Surgical interventions may be considered for individuals with severe OSA or anatomical abnormalities that contribute to airway obstruction. Surgical options may include procedures to remove excess tissue from the throat, reposition the jaw, or implant devices to support the soft palate and prevent airway collapse.

9. Weight Loss and Lifestyle Modifications: Weight loss and lifestyle modifications, such as regular exercise, dietary changes, and avoidance of alcohol and sedatives before bedtime, can help reduce excess weight and improve sleep apnea symptoms in some individuals.

10. Combination Therapies: Some individuals may benefit from combination therapies that incorporate elements of CPAP therapy with other treatment modalities, such as oral appliance therapy, positional therapy, or weight loss interventions. Combination therapies may offer synergistic effects and enhanced treatment outcomes for certain individuals.

When considering CPAP alternatives and variations, it's essential to consult with a healthcare provider or sleep specialist to determine the most appropriate treatment approach based on individual needs, preferences, and medical history. A comprehensive evaluation can help identify the most effective and suitable treatment options for managing obstructive sleep apnea and improving sleep quality and overall health.

Surgical Options for Snoring

- Types of Surgical Procedures Available:

1. Uvulopalatopharyngoplasty (UPPP): This procedure involves removing excess tissue from the uvula, soft palate, and throat to widen the airway and reduce vibration that causes snoring.

2. Tonsillectomy and Adenoidectomy: Surgical removal of enlarged tonsils and adenoids can alleviate airway obstruction and reduce snoring, especially in children and young adults.

3. Palatal Implants (Pillar Procedure): Small polyester implants are inserted into the soft palate to stiffen it, reducing tissue vibration and snoring.

4. Laser-Assisted Uvulopalatoplasty (LAUP): Laser energy is used to reshape and remove excess tissue from the uvula and soft palate, reducing airway obstruction and snoring.

5. Radiofrequency Ablation (RFA): This minimally invasive procedure uses radiofrequency energy to shrink and stiffen the soft palate, reducing tissue vibration and snoring.

6. Septoplasty and Turbinate Reduction: Surgery to correct a deviated septum or reduce the size of nasal turbinates can improve nasal airflow and reduce snoring caused by nasal obstruction.

- Risks and Benefits of Surgical Intervention:

- **Benefits:** Surgical procedures for snoring can effectively reduce or eliminate snoring in many cases, improving sleep quality for both the individual and their bed partner. Surgical intervention may also lead to improvements in daytime alertness, mood, and overall quality of life.

- **Risks:** Surgical procedures carry risks such as bleeding, infection, pain, swelling, and complications related to anesthesia. There is also a risk of recurrence of snoring or development of new symptoms post-surgery. Additionally, some surgical procedures may not be suitable for all individuals, and outcomes can vary depending on factors such as the underlying cause of snoring and individual anatomy.

- Considering Surgery as a Last Resort:

Surgery for snoring is typically considered as a last resort when conservative treatments, lifestyle modifications, and other interventions have failed to adequately control snoring or improve sleep quality. Before considering surgery, individuals should undergo a comprehensive evaluation by a healthcare provider or sleep specialist to determine the underlying cause of snoring and explore alternative treatment options.

It's essential to weigh the potential benefits and risks of surgical intervention carefully and have realistic expectations about the outcomes. Surgical procedures should only be pursued after thorough discussion with a healthcare provider, consideration of individual preferences and medical history, and understanding of the potential risks and benefits involved.

Surgical intervention may be recommended for individuals with severe snoring that significantly impacts their quality of life, disrupts their sleep or the sleep of their bed partner, and is associated with underlying health conditions such as obstructive sleep apnea. A multidisciplinary approach involving collaboration between healthcare providers, sleep specialists, and surgeons can help ensure comprehensive evaluation, personalized treatment planning, and optimal outcomes for individuals considering surgical intervention for snoring.

Seeking Professional Help

- Consulting with Sleep Specialists

Consulting with sleep specialists is an essential step in addressing and potentially curing snoring. Here's how consulting with sleep specialists can help:

1. Comprehensive Evaluation: Sleep specialists can conduct a comprehensive evaluation to determine the underlying cause of snoring. This evaluation may include a detailed medical history, physical examination, and possibly a sleep study (polysomnography) to assess sleep patterns, breathing, and potential sleep disorders such as obstructive sleep apnea (OSA).

2. Accurate Diagnosis: Sleep specialists can accurately diagnose the cause of snoring and identify any underlying sleep disorders or medical conditions contributing to the problem. An accurate diagnosis is essential for developing an effective treatment plan tailored to the individual's needs.

3. Personalized Treatment Plan: Based on the evaluation and diagnosis, sleep specialists can develop a personalized treatment plan to address snoring and any underlying sleep disorders or contributing factors. This treatment plan may include lifestyle modifications, behavioral changes, oral appliance therapy, CPAP therapy, surgery, or other interventions as appropriate.

4. Advanced Treatment Options: Sleep specialists can provide access to advanced treatment options for snoring, including specialized therapies such as oral appliance therapy, CPAP therapy, or surgical interventions. They can also offer guidance on the latest advancements in sleep medicine and technology to improve snoring and sleep quality.

5. Monitoring and Follow-Up: Sleep specialists can monitor progress and provide ongoing support and guidance throughout the treatment process. Regular follow-up appointments allow for adjustments to treatment as needed and ensure that the chosen interventions are effectively addressing snoring and improving sleep quality.

6. Multidisciplinary Approach: Sleep specialists often collaborate with other healthcare providers, including dentists, otolaryngologists (ear, nose, and throat specialists), pulmonologists, and psychologists, to provide comprehensive care for snoring and sleep disorders. A multidisciplinary approach ensures that all aspects of snoring and sleep health are addressed effectively.

7. Education and Support: Sleep specialists can educate individuals and their families about snoring, sleep disorders, treatment options, and lifestyle modifications to improve sleep quality and overall health. They can also provide support, resources, and guidance to help individuals navigate the challenges of managing snoring and sleep disorders.

By consulting with sleep specialists, individuals with snoring can receive expert evaluation, diagnosis, and treatment tailored to their specific needs, leading to improved sleep quality, better overall health, and potentially the cure of snoring.

- Participating in Sleep Studies

Participating in sleep studies can provide valuable insights into sleep patterns, breathing, and potential sleep disorders such as snoring and obstructive sleep apnea. Here's what you need to know about participating in sleep studies:

1. Consultation with a Sleep Specialist: Before participating in a sleep study, it's essential to consult with a sleep specialist or healthcare provider to determine if a sleep study is necessary and appropriate based on your symptoms, medical history, and risk factors for sleep disorders.

2. Types of Sleep Studies:
   - **Polysomnography (PSG):** PSG is a comprehensive sleep study conducted in a sleep laboratory or clinic overnight. It involves monitoring various physiological parameters during sleep, including brain waves, heart rate,

breathing patterns, muscle activity, and oxygen levels, to diagnose sleep disorders such as snoring, obstructive sleep apnea, central sleep apnea, insomnia, and restless legs syndrome.

- Home Sleep Apnea Testing (HSAT): HSAT is a simplified version of polysomnography that can be conducted at home. It typically measures breathing patterns, oxygen saturation, and airflow during sleep using portable monitoring devices. HSAT is often used to screen for obstructive sleep apnea in individuals with a high pre-test probability and no significant comorbidities.

3. Preparing for the Sleep Study:
 - Follow any pre-study instructions provided by the sleep specialist or sleep center, such as avoiding caffeine or certain medications before the study.
 - Bring comfortable sleepwear, toiletries, and any medications or

medical devices you may need during the study.

- Inform the sleep center staff of any specific concerns or preferences regarding the sleep study, such as sleeping habits, comfort preferences, or mobility issues.

4. During the Sleep Study:

- Arrive at the sleep center or laboratory at the scheduled time and follow the instructions provided by the staff.

- You will be fitted with sensors and monitoring equipment to measure various physiological parameters during sleep. These sensors are painless and non-invasive.

- Try to relax and sleep as naturally as possible during the study. The sleep technologist will monitor your sleep and assist you if needed.

5. After the Sleep Study:

- Once the sleep study is complete, you can typically return home and resume your normal activities.
- The data collected during the sleep study will be analyzed by a sleep specialist or healthcare provider to diagnose any sleep disorders and develop an appropriate treatment plan.
- Follow-up appointments may be scheduled to discuss the results of the sleep study, review treatment options, and address any questions or concerns you may have.

Participating in sleep studies can provide valuable information about your sleep patterns and help diagnose and manage sleep disorders such as snoring and obstructive sleep apnea. Working closely with a sleep specialist or healthcare provider ensures that you receive the appropriate evaluation, diagnosis, and treatment for your specific sleep concerns.

- Exploring Advanced Treatment Options

Exploring advanced treatment options for snoring and sleep disorders involves considering various interventions beyond lifestyle modifications and conservative therapies. Here are some advanced treatment options to explore:

1. Continuous Positive Airway Pressure (CPAP) Therapy:
   - CPAP therapy involves wearing a mask connected to a machine that delivers a continuous stream of air pressure to keep the airway open during sleep.
   - CPAP therapy is highly effective for treating obstructive sleep apnea (OSA) and reducing snoring associated with airway obstruction.
   - Advanced CPAP devices may offer features such as auto-adjusting pressure settings, heated humidification, and data tracking capabilities for improved comfort and compliance.

2. Bi-level Positive Airway Pressure (BiPAP) Therapy:

- BiPAP therapy delivers two levels of air pressure—one for inhalation and a lower pressure for exhalation—to assist individuals with breathing difficulties during sleep.

- BiPAP therapy may be beneficial for individuals with neuromuscular disorders, certain types of central sleep apnea, or those who have difficulty tolerating CPAP therapy.

3. Adaptive Servo-Ventilation (ASV) Therapy:

- ASV therapy is a specialized form of positive airway pressure therapy that adjusts the air pressure based on an individual's breathing patterns, providing a more customized and adaptive treatment approach.

- ASV therapy is often used for treating complex sleep apnea syndrome, central sleep apnea, or mixed sleep apnea.

4. Oral Appliance Therapy:

- Oral appliances are custom-fitted devices worn in the mouth during sleep to reposition the jaw and tongue, keeping the airway open and reducing snoring and sleep apnea events.

- Oral appliance therapy may be recommended for individuals with mild to moderate OSA or those who cannot tolerate CPAP therapy.

5. Inspire Therapy (Hypoglossal Nerve Stimulation):

- Inspire therapy is an implantable device that stimulates the hypoglossal nerve, which controls tongue movement, to prevent the collapse of the upper airway during sleep.

- Inspire therapy may be suitable for individuals with moderate to severe OSA who have not responded to other treatments and meet specific criteria for implantation.

6. Surgical Interventions:
 - Surgical procedures may be considered for individuals with severe snoring or sleep apnea who have not responded to conservative treatments.
 - Surgical options may include procedures such as uvulopalatopharyngoplasty (UPPP), tonsillectomy, adenoidectomy, maxillomandibular advancement (MMA) surgery, or hypoglossal nerve stimulation.

7. Nasal Valve Devices and Implants:
 - Nasal valve devices and implants are designed to improve nasal airflow and reduce nasal obstruction, which can contribute to snoring and sleep-disordered breathing.
 - These devices may be used as standalone treatments or in conjunction

with other therapies for snoring and sleep disorders.

When exploring advanced treatment options for snoring and sleep disorders, it's essential to consult with a sleep specialist or healthcare provider to determine the most appropriate treatment approach based on individual needs, preferences, and medical history. A comprehensive evaluation and personalized treatment plan ensure that individuals receive optimal care for their specific sleep concerns.

Coping Strategies for Partners

- _Understanding the Impact of Snoring on Relationships_

Snoring can have a significant impact on relationships, affecting both the snorer and their partner. Here's how snoring can affect relationships:

1. Sleep Disturbance: Snoring can disrupt the sleep of both the snorer and their partner, leading to sleep fragmentation, poor sleep quality, and daytime sleepiness. Sleep disturbances can strain the relationship and lead to irritability, moodiness, and difficulty concentrating during waking hours.

2. Bedroom Dynamics: Snoring may lead to changes in bedroom dynamics, such as separate sleeping arrangements or partners sleeping in different rooms to avoid the noise disturbance. While this may provide temporary relief from snoring, it can contribute to feelings of isolation, loneliness, and intimacy issues in the relationship.

3. **Resentment and Frustration:** Partners of snorers may experience feelings of resentment, frustration, or anger due to the constant disruption caused by snoring. Over time, unresolved issues related to snoring can escalate into conflicts and strain the emotional connection between partners.

4. **Communication Breakdown:** Snoring can interfere with effective communication between partners, especially if it leads to sleep deprivation, irritability, or mood swings. Poor communication can exacerbate relationship problems and make it challenging to address underlying issues related to snoring and sleep disturbances.

5. Sexual Intimacy: Sleep disturbances caused by snoring can impact sexual intimacy and desire, leading to decreased libido and relationship dissatisfaction. Fatigue, irritability, and decreased arousal associated with poor sleep quality may affect sexual performance and satisfaction for both partners.

6. Health Concerns: Chronic snoring may be a sign of underlying sleep disorders such as obstructive sleep apnea (OSA), which can have serious health consequences if left untreated. Partners may worry about the snorer's health and well-being, leading to increased stress and anxiety in the relationship.

7. Support and Understanding: Partners of snorers may feel torn between the desire to support their loved one and the need for quality sleep. Finding a balance between providing support and addressing sleep disturbances can be challenging and may require open communication, empathy, and compromise from both partners.

8. Seeking Solutions Together: Addressing snoring and sleep disturbances as a couple can strengthen the relationship and foster a sense of teamwork and mutual support. Exploring treatment options, seeking medical advice, and implementing lifestyle changes together can demonstrate commitment to improving sleep health and relationship dynamics.

Overall, snoring can impact relationships in various ways, affecting sleep quality, emotional well-being, and intimacy between partners. Addressing snoring and sleep disturbances requires patience, understanding, and a willingness to work together as a couple to find effective solutions and maintain a healthy and fulfilling relationship.

- *Communication Techniques for Addressing Snoring Concerns*

Addressing snoring concerns requires open and empathetic communication between partners. Here are some communication techniques for discussing snoring concerns in a constructive and supportive manner:

1. Choose the Right Time and Place: Pick a time when both partners are relaxed and free from distractions to have a conversation about snoring. Avoid discussing sensitive topics when one partner is stressed, tired, or busy with other responsibilities.

2. Express Concerns with Empathy: Start the conversation by expressing your concerns about the impact of snoring on both partners' sleep and overall well-being. Use "I" statements to communicate how the snoring affects you personally without placing blame on your partner.

3. **Focus on the Behavior, Not the Person:** When discussing snoring, focus on the behavior itself rather than criticizing or blaming your partner. Emphasize that snoring is a common issue that many people experience and that you want to work together to find a solution.

4. **Listen Actively:** Listen to your partner's perspective without interrupting or becoming defensive. Show empathy and understanding towards their feelings and concerns about snoring. Acknowledge their experiences and validate their emotions to create a supportive atmosphere for discussion.

5. **Offer Encouragement and Support:** Offer reassurance to your partner that you are committed to finding a solution

to the snoring issue together. Encourage them to seek medical evaluation and explore treatment options for snoring or sleep disorders. Provide support and encouragement throughout the process of addressing snoring concerns.

6. Brainstorm Solutions Together: Collaborate with your partner to brainstorm potential solutions for addressing snoring, such as lifestyle changes, sleeping arrangements, or seeking medical advice. Explore different treatment options and discuss the pros and cons of each approach to find the best fit for both partners.

7. Be Patient and Flexible: Addressing snoring concerns may require time, patience, and experimentation with different strategies and interventions. Be patient with each other as you navigate the process of finding effective solutions. Stay flexible and open-minded to adjusting your approach based on feedback and outcomes.

8. **Seek Professional Guidance if Needed:** If snoring persists despite efforts to address it at home, consider seeking professional guidance from a sleep specialist or healthcare provider. A sleep specialist can conduct a thorough evaluation, diagnose any underlying sleep disorders, and recommend appropriate treatment options tailored to your individual needs.

By using these communication techniques, couples can discuss snoring concerns openly and collaboratively, fostering a supportive and understanding environment for finding effective solutions and improving sleep quality for both partners.

- Seeking Support and Resources for Partners

Seeking support and resources for partners affected by snoring can help them navigate the challenges and find effective solutions. Here are some ways partners can seek support and access helpful resources:

1. Educate Yourself: Partners can educate themselves about snoring, its causes, and potential treatment options. Understanding the underlying factors contributing to snoring can help partners support each other and explore appropriate interventions together.

2. Encourage Open Communication: Partners can encourage open communication about snoring concerns and their impact on both individuals' sleep quality and overall well-being. Create a safe and supportive space for discussing snoring issues, feelings, and concerns without judgment or criticism.

3. Join Support Groups: Partners can seek support from online or in-person support groups for individuals affected by snoring or sleep disorders. Support groups provide opportunities to connect with others who are experiencing similar challenges, share experiences, and exchange advice and coping strategies.

4. Attend Couples Counseling: Couples counseling can help partners address communication difficulties, resolve conflicts related to snoring, and strengthen their relationship. A qualified therapist can facilitate productive discussions, promote understanding and empathy, and assist couples in finding mutually acceptable solutions to snoring concerns.

5. Explore Treatment Options Together: Partners can explore treatment options for snoring and sleep disorders together, including lifestyle changes, medical interventions, and alternative therapies. Consult with healthcare providers or sleep specialists to discuss potential treatment approaches and develop a personalized plan that meets both partners' needs and preferences.

6. **Support Healthy Lifestyle Changes:** Partners can support each other in making healthy lifestyle changes that may help reduce snoring, such as maintaining a healthy weight, avoiding alcohol and sedatives before bedtime, practicing good sleep hygiene, and establishing a consistent sleep schedule.

7. **Seek Professional Guidance:** Partners affected by snoring can seek professional guidance from healthcare providers or sleep specialists. A qualified healthcare provider can conduct a comprehensive evaluation,

diagnose any underlying sleep disorders, and recommend appropriate treatment options tailored to individual needs.

8. Use Technology and Apps: Partners can use technology and smartphone apps designed to monitor snoring patterns, track sleep quality, and provide personalized feedback and recommendations for improving sleep habits. These tools can help partners better understand their sleep patterns and monitor progress over time.

By seeking support and accessing resources, partners affected by snoring can find effective ways to address snoring concerns, improve sleep quality, and strengthen their relationship. Working together as a team and supporting each other through the process can lead to positive outcomes and a healthier, happier partnership.

Long-Term Maintenance and Prevention

- *Monitoring Snoring Patterns Over Time*

Monitoring snoring patterns over time can provide valuable insights into the severity and frequency of snoring episodes, as well as the effectiveness of interventions and treatments. Here's how to monitor snoring patterns over time:

1. Keep a Snoring Diary: Start by keeping a snoring diary to track snoring episodes over a period of time, such as several weeks or months. Note the date, time, duration, and intensity of each snoring episode, as well as any factors that may contribute to snoring, such as sleeping position, alcohol consumption, or nasal congestion.

2. Use Snoring Apps or Devices: Consider using smartphone apps or wearable devices designed to monitor snoring patterns during sleep. These apps and devices typically use microphone or accelerometer technology to detect snoring sounds or movements and provide data on snoring frequency, duration, and intensity.

3. Consult with a Sleep Specialist: If snoring persists or worsens over time, consult with a sleep specialist or healthcare provider for a comprehensive evaluation. A sleep specialist can conduct a thorough assessment, diagnose any underlying sleep disorders contributing to snoring, and recommend appropriate treatment options based on individual needs.

4. Undergo Sleep Studies: In some cases, a sleep study (polysomnography) may be recommended to evaluate snoring patterns and assess sleep quality. During a sleep study, various physiological parameters are monitored overnight to detect sleep disorders such as obstructive sleep apnea (OSA) and identify factors contributing to snoring.

5. Implement Lifestyle Changes: Make lifestyle changes to reduce snoring and improve sleep quality over time. This may include maintaining a healthy weight, avoiding alcohol and sedatives before bedtime, practicing good sleep hygiene, and establishing a consistent sleep schedule.

6. Monitor Treatment Effectiveness: If you undergo treatment for snoring or sleep disorders, monitor the effectiveness of the treatment over time. Keep track of any changes in snoring patterns, sleep quality, and daytime symptoms after initiating treatment, and communicate with your healthcare provider or sleep specialist about any concerns or improvements.

7. Adjust Interventions as Needed: Based on monitoring snoring patterns and treatment effectiveness over time, adjust interventions as needed to optimize outcomes. This may involve modifying lifestyle factors, trying different treatment modalities, or seeking additional support and guidance from healthcare providers.

By monitoring snoring patterns over time and adjusting interventions as needed, individuals can gain a better understanding of their sleep habits, identify factors contributing to snoring, and make informed decisions about managing snoring and improving sleep quality for the long term.

- Incorporating Healthy Habits into Your Lifestyle

Incorporating healthy habits into your lifestyle can help reduce snoring and improve overall sleep quality. Here are some key habits to consider:

1. Maintain a Healthy Weight: Excess weight, especially around the neck and throat, can contribute to airway obstruction and snoring. Aim to maintain a healthy weight through a balanced diet and regular exercise.

2. Avoid Alcohol and Sedatives Before Bed: Alcohol and sedatives can relax the muscles in the throat and tongue, leading to increased snoring and sleep disturbances. Avoid consuming alcohol or sedatives close to bedtime.

3. Practice Good Sleep Hygiene: Establish a regular sleep schedule and bedtime routine to promote better sleep quality. Create a relaxing environment in your bedroom, limit exposure to screens before bedtime, and avoid stimulating activities that can interfere with sleep.

4. Sleep on Your Side: Sleeping on your back can exacerbate snoring by causing the tongue and soft tissues in the throat to collapse backward. Try sleeping on your side to keep the airway open and reduce snoring.

5. Elevate Your Head: Elevating the head of your bed or using extra pillows to elevate your head can help reduce snoring by opening up the airway and promoting better breathing during sleep.

6. Stay Hydrated: Drink plenty of water throughout the day to stay hydrated. Dehydration can lead to thicker mucus in the throat, which can exacerbate snoring.

7. Manage Nasal Congestion: Address nasal congestion or allergies that can contribute to snoring by using saline nasal sprays, nasal decongestants, or allergy medications as needed.

8. Quit Smoking: Smoking irritates the throat and airways, leading to inflammation and increased mucus production, which can contribute to snoring. Quitting smoking can improve overall respiratory health and reduce snoring.

9. Exercise Regularly: Engage in regular physical activity to improve overall health and reduce the risk of snoring. Exercise can help strengthen muscles in the throat and promote better breathing during sleep.

10. Manage Stress: Stress and anxiety can negatively impact sleep quality and contribute to snoring. Practice relaxation techniques such as deep breathing, meditation, or yoga to reduce stress and promote better sleep.

Incorporating these healthy habits into your lifestyle can help reduce snoring, improve sleep quality, and enhance overall well-being. Consistency and perseverance are key, so make small changes gradually and prioritize habits that support better sleep hygiene and respiratory health. If snoring persists despite lifestyle modifications, consider seeking guidance from a healthcare provider or sleep specialist for further evaluation and treatment.

- *Staying Informed about Advances in Snoring Treatment*

Staying informed about advances in snoring treatment can help individuals access the latest interventions and make informed decisions about managing their snoring. Here are some ways to stay informed:

1. Research and Education: Stay updated on the latest research, studies, and advancements in snoring treatment by reading reputable sources such as medical journals, research articles, and healthcare websites. Look for information from trusted organizations and institutions specializing in sleep medicine and respiratory health.

2. Consult with Healthcare Providers: Regularly consult with healthcare providers, including primary care physicians, sleep specialists, and otolaryngologists (ear, nose, and throat specialists), to discuss new developments in snoring treatment and explore appropriate interventions based on individual needs and preferences.

3. Attend Seminars and Workshops: Attend seminars, workshops, or conferences on sleep medicine and respiratory health to learn about emerging trends, innovative therapies, and best practices in snoring treatment. These events often feature presentations by leading experts and researchers in the field.

4. Join Support Groups: Join online or in-person support groups for individuals affected by snoring or sleep disorders. These support groups provide opportunities to connect with others who are experiencing similar challenges, share experiences, and exchange information about treatment options and resources.

5. **Follow Healthcare Organizations:** Follow healthcare organizations, professional societies, and advocacy groups specializing in sleep medicine and respiratory health on social media platforms or subscribe to their newsletters to receive updates on advancements in snoring treatment, research findings, and educational resources.

6. **Stay Informed About New Technologies:** Stay informed about new technologies and devices designed to diagnose and treat snoring, such as wearable sleep trackers, smartphone apps, and medical devices. Explore how

these technologies can be integrated into your snoring management plan and discuss them with your healthcare provider.

7. Participate in Clinical Trials: Consider participating in clinical trials or research studies investigating novel treatments for snoring and sleep disorders. Clinical trials provide opportunities to access cutting-edge therapies and contribute to the advancement of medical knowledge in the field of sleep medicine.

8. Engage with Online Communities: Engage with online communities, forums, and discussion groups focused on snoring treatment and sleep health. Participate in discussions, ask questions, and share experiences with others who are seeking information and support related to snoring management.

By staying informed about advances in snoring treatment, individuals can access the latest interventions, make informed decisions about their healthcare, and take proactive steps to manage their snoring and improve sleep quality. Remember to consult with healthcare providers for personalized guidance and recommendations tailored to your specific needs and circumstances.

Conclusion

As we draw to a close in our exploration of snoring and its remedies, it's evident that the journey to peaceful sleep involves understanding, commitment, and a multifaceted approach. Throughout this book, we've delved into the intricacies of snoring, its causes, and its effects on our health and relationships. From recognizing the severity of our snoring to seeking professional evaluation, we've taken the first crucial steps towards reclaiming restful nights.

In the realm of lifestyle changes, we've uncovered the power of simple yet effective habits. Improving sleep hygiene, maintaining a consistent sleep schedule, and creating a calming bedtime routine have emerged as pillars of healthy sleep habits. By optimizing our sleep environment and making mindful dietary choices, we not only address snoring but also enhance overall well-being.

The chapters on avoiding alcohol and sedatives shed light on substances that can exacerbate snoring, offering strategies to reduce dependency and promote better sleep quality. Practical techniques such as positional therapy, nasal congestion relief, and throat exercises provide actionable steps to alleviate snoring and improve airflow during sleep. By incorporating daily exercise routines and exploring devices like oral appliances and CPAP therapy, we widen our arsenal against snoring.

For those considering surgical options, we've outlined the types of procedures available, along with their risks and benefits, emphasizing surgery as a last resort. Seeking professional help, whether through consultations with sleep specialists or participation in sleep studies, opens doors to advanced treatment options tailored to individual needs.

Recognizing the impact of snoring on relationships, we've explored coping strategies for partners, emphasizing communication and support as keys to navigating this common issue together. Looking towards the future, we've discussed the importance of long-term maintenance and prevention, advocating for the monitoring of snoring patterns over time and the incorporation of healthy habits into our lifestyles.

As we bid farewell to these pages, let us remember that the journey to overcoming snoring is not a solitary one. It's a journey that requires patience, perseverance, and a willingness to explore various avenues until we find what works best for us. With each chapter, we've equipped ourselves with knowledge and tools to embark on this journey with confidence.

So, here's to quieter nights and rejuvenating sleep. May the insights gained from these pages serve as guiding lights, leading us towards the restful slumber we deserve. As we embrace healthier habits and stay informed about advances in snoring treatment, let us pave the way for a future filled with tranquil nights and revitalized mornings. Goodbye, and may your nights be filled with peaceful silence.

If you found this book to be an engaging and enriching experience, your feedback is invaluable. Leaving a review on Amazon not only supports me as a writer but also aids fellow readers in making informed decisions. Your review provides crucial insights that guide my growth as a writer, allowing me to refine my craft and deliver even more better books in the future. Your words have the power to shape the reading experiences of others, ensuring they discover books that resonate with them. Take a moment to share your thoughts on Amazon, and together, let's enrich the literary community one review at a time.

www.ingramcontent.com/pod-product-compliance
Lightning Source LLC
Chambersburg PA
CBHW052249220526
45471CB00001B/259